To Nancy

It has been a pleasure knowing you

Eleni Delfakis

Healthy Living From A Greek Island

How To Achieve Good Health &
Enjoy What You Eat

Loose Weight
Look Great
Live Longer

NUTRITION GUIDE & COOKBOOK

WRITTEN BY

Eleni Delfakis, M.S., R.D.

COPPER HILL PRESS
TUCSON, ARIZONA
U.S.A

Healthy Living From A Greek Island

How to Achieve Good Health & Enjoy What You Eat

By Eleni Delfakis, M.S., R.D.

Published by:
Copper Hill Press
Post Office Box 13628
Tucson, Arizona 85732-3628
http://www.copperhillpress.com

Cover Art by Konstantina A. Delfakis

All rights reserved. No part of this book may be reproduced or transmitted in any form or by any means, without the written permission from the author.

Copyright 2003, Eleni Delfakis

ISBN: 0-9724038-9-2
First Printing 2003

Library of Congress Cataloging-in-Publication Data

Delfakis, Eleni
  Healthy living from a Greek island : how to achieve good health & enjoy what you eat : nutrition guide & cookbook/written by Eleni Delfakis, -- 1st ed.
  p. cm.
  Includes bibliographical references and index.
  LCCN: 2002113087
  ISBN: 0972403892

  1. Nutrition. 2. Health. 3. Obesity—United States. 4. Cookery, Greek. I. Title.

RA784.D45 2003   613.2
                        QBI02-200711

CONTENTS

ABOUT THE AUTHOR	ix
A NOTE TO THE READER	x
ACKNOWLEDGEMENTS	xi
INTRODUCTION	xii

CHAPTER

1 URGENT NEED TO CHANGE THE WAY WE LIVE   1

What Is Obesity?	1
Types Of Body Fat	3
How to Measure Your BMR	4
Preventable Diseases	5
Recent Changes in the Food Supply & American Preferences	10
Current Lifestyle Trends	14
Osteoporosis	16
Risk Factors for Osteoporosis	17
The Importance of Calcium in the Diet	18

2 CURRENT FOOD TRENDS AMONG OUR CHILDREN   27

Major Factors Contributing to Childhood Obesity	30
Healthy Food Habits for the Whole Family	32
Behavior Modification for Small Children	33
Healthy Snacks	34
Dietary Recommendations for Children Age 2-12	35
Dietary Recommendations for Teenagers	36

| 3 | **OUR NUTRIENT REQUIREMENTS** | 37 |

    Energy Needs   37
    Carbohydrates and Protein   40
    Fats
    Vitamins   45
    Minerals and Trace Elements   48
    Phytochemicals and Antioxidants   52
    Special Nutritional Needs for Older Adults   53
    Nourish the Skin from With-in   55
    Relief from Allergies   57

| 4 | **BALANCE YOUR DIET** | 61 |

    How to Start Living Healthier   61
    Fifteen Steps To Optimal Health   63
    Foods That Fight Against Diseases & Aging   65
    Daily Meal Plan   74

| 5 | **PORTIONS SIZES** | 76 |

    What is a Portion?   76
    Food Serving Portion Charts   81

| 6 | **THE BENEFITS OF LIVING AN ACTIVE LIFE** | 91 |

    Aerobic & Anaerobic Activities   93
    Muscle Fitness   93
    Proper Hydration   94
    Relaxation   94
    Height & Weight Chart for Women   97
    Height & Weight Chart for Men   98
    To Determine Your Calorie Needs   99

COOKBOOK   101

| 7 | **BASIC INGREDIENTS & FOOD SAFETY** | 102 |

	Basic ingredients	102
	Food born Illness	110
	Handling Seafood	111
	Handling Poultry & Eggs	113
	Tips for Safe Food Handling	114
8	**STARTERS & VEGETARIAN DISHES**	**115**
	Hardy White Bread	116
	Pita Bread	117
	Zucchini Omelet	118
	Greek Salad	119
	Pepper and Peach Salad	120
	Village Salad	121
	Winter Salad	122
	Eggplant Salad	123
	Potato Salad	124
	Chicken Salad	125
	Lentil Soup	126
	Chicken Lemon Soup	127
	Bean Soup	129
	Potato Clam Soup	130
	Cheese Puffs	131
	Egg Whites Stuffed With Liver Pate	133
	Sautéed Calamari	134
	Sautéed Meatballs	135
	Zucchini Croquettes	136
	Stuffed Grape Leaves	137
	Yogurt & Cucumber Sauce	138
	Yellow Split Pea Spread	139
	Red Roasted Peppers Stuffed with Cheese	140
	Cheese Spread with Smoked Salmon	141
9	**VEGETARIAN DISHES**	**142**
	Pita Stuffed with Avocado Salad	143
	Portabella Mushroom Sandwich	144
	Black-eyed Peas with Rice	145
	Green Beans with Tomatoes & Herbs	146
	Fettuccine with Garlic & Basil	147
	Risotto with Spinach	148

	Artichokes & Potatoes in Lemon Sauce	149
	Garlic Mashed Potatoes	150
	Baked Beans	151
	Seared Vegetables	152
	Rice Pilaf	153
	Steamed Greens	154
	Eggplant Vinaigrette	155
	Spinach with Peppers & Almonds	156
	Tomatoes Stuffed with Rice & Herbs	157
	Spinach & Cheese Pie	158
	Potatoes with Green Peas	160
	Potatoes with Oregano & Lemon	161
	Butter Beans with Dill	161
10	**MEAT & POULTRY DISHES**	**162**
	Lamb Chops with Mushrooms & Mint	163
	Braised Lamb in Red Wine Sauce	164
	Lamb with Pine Nuts & Raisings	165
	Roast Lamb & Potatoes	166
	Pork Tenderloin with Apples & Apricots	167
	Baked Italian Meatballs	168
	Veal Scaloppini	169
	Baked Ziti with Meat Sauce	170
	Spanish Salsa	171
	Chicken Enchiladas	172
	Green Chile Sauce	173
	Beef Burritos with Green Chile Sauce	174
	Oriental Chicken & Shrimp	175
	Roast Chicken & Potatoes	176
	Roast Cornish Hens with Apples & Raisins	177
	Chicken with Herbs and Wine	178
11	**SEAFOOD DISHES**	**179**
	Baked Clams	180
	Shrimp with Garlic & Feta	181
	Chilled Shrimp & Crab Salad	182
	Baked Filet of Halibut	183
	Filet Of Sole with Almonds	183
	Mussels in Red Wine Sauce	185

	Seafood Chowder	186
	Baked Salmon	187
	Belgium Endives Stuffed with Salmon	188
	Salmon Glazed with Honey & Almonds	189
	Sea-Bass and Scallops in White Wine Sauce	191
	Baked Trout	192
12	**THE SWEETS SHOP**	**193**
	Baklava	194
	Butter Cookies	196
	Honey Macaroons	197
	Apples Baked in Phyllo Pastry	199
	Rice Pudding	200
	Spanish Custard	201
	Semolina Custard with Raspberries	202
	Walnut Cake	203
	Yogurt Cake	204
	Bread Pudding	205
	Crepes with Yogurt & Fresh Berries	206
	Donut Puffs with Honey & Nuts	207
	Easter Bread	208
	Banana & Zucchini Bread	209
	New Year's Day Cake	210
HERBAL REMEDIES, ALCOHOL & CAFFEINE CONSUMPTION		**211**
13	**HERBAL REMEDIES**	**212**
	Popular Herbal Remedies	214
	Dangerous Herbs	219
14	**THE FACTS ABOUT ALCOHOL**	**223**
	How much is Moderate Drinking?	227
	How much is One Drink?	228
	Who Should Not Consume Alcohol	228
	Wines from Greece	229

15	**CAFFEINE**	230
	Coffee	230
	Coffee Consumption in Relation To Health & Disease	232
	Guidelines for Coffee Drinkers	235
	Tea	235
	The Benefits of Tea Consumption	238
	Suggestions for Tea Drinkers	238
GLOSSARY		239
REFERENCES		243
INDEX		251

About The Author

Eleni Delfakis, M.S., R.D. earned a Masters of Science in Dietetics with an emphasis in nutrition education from The University of Arizona. In addition, she has earned her dietetic credentials and membership from the American Dietetics Association. She enjoyed success as an educator, owner and chef of an award-winning restaurant in Tucson, and is a co-author of a food service textbook and teacher's manual.

Eleni Delfakis is native to the Greek island of Crete where her parents and countless generations of her family were born. She currently resides in Tucson, Arizona and maintains the healthy lifestyle that is characteristic of her beautiful home island. "Healthy Living from A Greek Island" reflects the culmination of Ms. Delfakis' widely recognized expertise in nutrition, food service, and from the vast richness of her home island's unique culture.

NOTE TO THE READER

The statistics of obesity in the United States, as well as around the world, have reached an all-time high. Over sixty percent of American adults are currently overweight with equally alarming rates among our children. Over the last three decades, a plethora of research shows that being overweight contributes to the risk of heart disease, diabetes, hypertension, as well as some types of cancer. The above statistics leave us with only one option; we must change the way we live today!

This book is a nutrition guide for the whole family. It outlines the reasons why we are overweight and what we can do about it, including research on herbal remedies, alcohol, caffeine, and how their consumption affects our health. In addition, the cookbook section will provide you with healthy and delicious recipes.

If you are interested being healthy and looking your best, without compromising good taste, <u>this book is for you!</u>

Acknowledgments

I am dedicating this book to my father's memory, a wonderful father and a great chef who loved to cook, and modeled good health habits for his children. He was the inspiration and strength behind every important decision in my life, including my love for nutrition and cooking.

Thank you Dad,

Eleni Delfakis, M.S., R.D.

INTRODUCTION

The essence of a good life is health, love and prosperity. Good health is a priority because without it, we will not enjoy the other two. However, while the foodservice industry has prospered over the last four decades, Americans are getting heavier, and the incidence of death from heart disease and diabetes are on the rise. The great majority of us do not exercise regularly and over forty percent do not exercise at all. The latest statistics reveal that sixty-one percent of the adult population in the U.S. is overweight or obese, with related healthcare costs exceeding 115 billions dollars annually. We are an unhealthy society and in addition, we are paying more for it in healthcare, diet aids and many other related costs. In June 2002, President George W. Bush launched the "Healthier U.S." initiative, the revival of the President's Council on Physical Fitness, and emphasized the importance of diet and exercise for all Americans.

To make things worse, over twenty-five percent of children under the age of eighteen are either overweight or obese. In the U.S. alone, over 300,000 people die every year from overweight related diseases, making obesity the second leading cause of preventable deaths; smoking is number one. The U.S. Surgeon General warns that obesity may soon become the number one preventable death, if we fail to treat this threat with greater awareness and urgency. These findings reach across the country and include people at all socioeconomic levels. The World

Health Organization has declared obesity "one of the greatest neglected public health problems of our time." People are not living to their fullest due to pain and suffering from illness. The majority of deaths are due to diseases that are preventable such as diabetes, heart disease, cancer and osteoporosis. The current dietary patterns are a threat to public health and can lead to serious physical and mental problems. This provides evidence that only a few among us are eating healthy.

How did the most sophisticated, best-educated and affluent nation in the world become obese and why? Aggressive marketing combined with a decline of home food preparation has led to bad eating habits. Schools offer our children and young adults primarily unhealthy foods, and not all teach the importance of nutrition and exercise. Dietary staples for most students from kindergarten to college include burgers, fries, pizza, soda, candy bars and ice cream. Most college students gain excessive weight the first year away from home. A large burger, large fries, and large soft drink can total up to 2,000 calories with half of the calories derived from fat. Furthermore, the same unhealthy foods permeate our presence, being readily available in movie theaters, sporting events and most other social venues of activity.

In our struggle to look great we have shifted from healthy eating to problem treating. We want our food experiences to be simple and entertaining, however, we are simply eating too much food. Research shows that in the past twenty years most of the health problems were due to eating too many calories from fat and refined sugars, over-consumption of salt, and not enough vegetables, fruit or whole grains and fiber. It is apparent that a good majority of us are not healthy and the future does not look very promising unless we change our lifestyle and the way we eat. It is time to consider where we are headed in terms of health and longevity.

An example of a population group well known among researchers, and who have long practiced healthy eating habits, are the people on the island of Crete, Greece. Since my parents were born and raised on the island, I have personally experienced the lifestyle and eating habits during my own childhood, as well as during my annual visits to the island as an adult. Their diet is unique and simple; it consists of a variety of foods flavored with a careful selection of fresh herbs and olive oil. In addition, most of the foods consumed are primarily from fresh sources; not from precooked, canned or processed.

My book offers long-term solutions to the current problems that prevent us from achieving optimal health. I do not offer "quick fix" answers. However, if you follow my suggestions you will improve your health, look and feel your best, and additionally; you will learn how to prepare delicious meals and enjoy what you eat.

CHAPTER 1

URGENT NEED TO CHANGE THE WAY WE LIVE

WHAT IS OBESITY?

Obesity is defined as excess accumulation of body fat tissue above and beyond the acceptable levels. This excess fat accumulates when calorie intake is greater than calorie expenditure for weight and height. There are two types of obesity: <u>endogenous obesity</u> caused by genetic and hormonal factors, and <u>exogenous obesity</u> caused by environmental and behavioral factors. Overweight and obese people are at risk for heart disease, hypertension, diabetes, gallbladder disease, stroke and some types of cancer. Obese children are at risk for respiratory problems, high blood pressure, elevated cholesterol and heart disease at a very young age. The majority of obese adults have <u>at least one</u> of the following conditions: diabetes, high blood pressure, and elevated blood cholesterol.

Only a small percent of obesity cases today can be attributed to heredity. Most experts agree that genetics may determine a person's frame size and body type, but current statistics in child and adult obesity cannot be blamed on genetics. Less than ten percent of all the childhood obesity cases are due to genetic factors. Other factors include ethnicity, gender, metabolic rate, hormone levels, diet, physical activity and weather. All of these factors contribute to the onset of the disease at an early age or later in life. However, a child born to two biological parents who are obese is more likely to become obese. Childhood obesity often persists to adulthood.

Overweight people die younger from diseases and post-surgical complications. In addition, they tend to suffer from arthritis in the knees, hips and lower spine, swelling of the legs and varicose veins. Obese people also suffer from social and economic disadvantages, such as humiliation by peers, discrimination in the job market, difficulties in traveling, in dating or maintaining relationships, and also pay higher insurance rates. These social and economic factors make obesity a handicap and a source of great emotional stress, which often leads to further increase in weight, as people respond to complex human sensations such as cravings, addictions, compulsions and yearnings. A person who is emotionally insecure about being accepted by others may indulge in eating to substitute for the love or friendship he/she seeks. Some researchers believe that overeating may be helping people escape depression.

A stressful lifestyle, with which most of us identify, also adds to the problem of obesity. When a person is stressed, a physiological response releases a hormone (cortisol), which initiates a desire to eat high fat and high sugar foods. Starvation and strict dieting induces a self-imposed stress and consequent weight gain, including a constant preoccupation with food and eating. To further complicate the problem of obesity, our society has very little compassion for fat people. They are often blamed for having no will power, for being lazy and for not caring. We have more compassion for people who smoke or abuse drugs or alcohol. However, when it comes to food related problems most people have no compassion or understand the magnitude of the problem; we must change this as a society, and be proactive and supportive.

TYPES OF BODY FAT

The two types of fat that characterize body fat are <u>hyper-tropic</u> and <u>hyper-cellular</u>. Hyper-tropic fat is characterized by enlarged fat cells and increased abdominal fat, resulting in the "apple shape." People with this type of fat have greater risks for developing hypertension and heart disease. Hyper-cellular fat is characterized by an increase in the number of fat cells, resulting in fat throughout the body. This type of fat is partly inherited, difficult to treat, and strongly influenced by diet and exercise. Once the fat cells increase in number, it becomes a lifelong struggle to keep the weight off.

Once a person becomes overweight, it is not easy to lose the weight. Enlarged fat cells for example, are insulin resistant (insulin is the hormone that promotes the uptake of glucose by the cells and its conversion to fat); therefore, the excess glucose remains in the blood stimulating the pancreas to *produce more insulin. This process promotes the storage of more fat. To further complicate things, the enlarged fat cells are not sensitive to hormones that promote fat breakdown. This is why it is much easier to prevent obesity rather than to treat it. Clinicians use the Body Mass Index (BMI) to estimate a person's body fat status. The BMI = weight in kilograms divided by height squared. However, this tool cannot be used for athletes or body builders because muscle is heavier than fat, and since they have a high proportion of muscle mass they tend to weigh more.*

How To Determine Your Body Mass Index (BMI)

Example: Calculate the BMI for a woman who stands 5'6" and weighs 140 lbs

Step 1.   140lbs divided by 2.2 lb/kg = 63.6 kg

Step 2.   5'6" = 66 inches divided by 40 inches in 1 meter = 1.65 meters.

Step 3.   Height Squared = 1.65 X 1.65 = 2.72

Step 4.   BMI = 63.6 divided by 2.72 = 23.4

BODY MASS INDEX (BMI) TABLE

Body Fat Status	BMI
Underweight	<18.5
Normal weight	<25
Overweight	25-29.9
Stage I Obesity	30-34.9
Stage II Obesity	35-39.9
Stage III Obesity	≥ 40

PREVENTABLE DISEASES

CANCER

Cancer is the second leading cause of death. While a large percentage of the population knows that obesity causes diabetes, hypertension and heart disease, only a small percentage know that it can also cause cancer. According to the American Institute of Cancer Research obesity is associated with colon, breast and other types of cancer. Cancer develops when something in the cells causes damage to the cell, resulting in the birth of a new mutated cell that is abnormal. These abnormal cells divide and multiply to form a tumor. If the cells in the tumor are able to escape, they can spread the cancer to other parts of the body. For the last two decades researchers have known that Src, a protein, was responsible in cancer metastasis, but they did not know how it was done. However, new research reveals that Src influences cell metastasis by loosening the tissue around the tumor to become porous and allow the cancer cells to escape to other parts of the body.

Strong evidence suggests that 40% of all the cancers could be prevented by a healthy diet and exercise, especially among people who eat a lot of vegetables and fruits, and consume very small amounts of animal fat. Therefore, maintaining ideal body weight, eating a healthy diet, living an active life, eliminating stress and not smoking is the best way we have in fighting against this monster of a disease.

HEART DISEASE

Atherosclerosis is a disease caused by an accumulation of fatty deposits inside the artery walls, which increases the risk of heart disease. Heart disease is the number one killer in most developed countries around the world, causing more than 500,000 deaths annually. Although there are many factors involved in developing heart disease, dietary cholesterol and obesity are leading causes. Cholesterol is a waxy substance that is manufactured in small amounts by the liver. It is carried to and from the body organs in fat and protein structures. Low-density lipoproteins [LDL], bad cholesterol, deliver cholesterol to the organs and arteries; and, high-density lipoproteins [HDL], good cholesterol, carry the excess away. High levels of the LDL in the blood is considered harmful because they are stored in the body tissues and arteries, while the HDL helps to protect the cells from fatty deposits. Cholesterol is necessary for many body functions, but too much forms fatty plaque deposits on the walls of blood vessels, causing loss of elasticity, narrowing and clogging. This condition is called atherosclerosis. If the arteries carrying the blood to the heart are blocked, the blockage causes a heart attack. If the arteries that carry blood to the brain are clogged, it causes a stroke.

Foods that are high in saturated fat, both from animal and vegetable sources, elevate cholesterol levels in the blood. Most of our favorite foods are hidden sources of saturated fats such as dairy products, fried foods, fast foods, cookies, crackers and non-dairy creamers. Foods that are high in cholesterol include egg yolks, animal organs, meat and poultry fat. Controlling the amount and type of fat consumed is important in lowering the risk of heart disease, stroke and cancer.

The blood level of cholesterol is under control naturally when we eat a healthy diet and live an active life. The human body has the ability to monitor the production of cholesterol so that when you eat more cholesterol, the body's metabolism produces less to keep the amount needed constant. If we eat less, our body will produce more to make up for the deficit. Too much saturated fat in the diet can contribute to high levels of cholesterol in the blood. However, some dietary fat is necessary to help absorb and transport important fat-soluble vitamins, and perform other metabolic processes. The question is how much? An overwhelming number of research studies show that monounsaturated fats, such as olive oil, protect the arteries from plaque by maintaining a healthy level of cholesterol in the blood. On the other hand, consuming foods containing high amounts of saturated fat contributes to fatty waste deposits in the arteries and blocks antioxidant reactions. I will discuss dietary fat in chapter three. The following list of foods are high in saturated fat, and if consumed frequently, cause clogging of the arteries, block antioxidant reactions and contribute to heart disease.

- Fatty meats
- Organ meats
- Bread made from animal fat
- Whole milk
- Commercial mixes
- Lard
- Coconut Oil
- Bacon
- Commercially fried foods
- Trans Fats (hydrogenated margarine, shortening)

Diabetes

Diabetes is a metabolic disease characterized by an insufficient supply of effective insulin, which renders the body unable to regulate blood glucose. Overeating and sedentary lifestyle are largely responsible for the current and alarming incidence of diabetes. Over twenty million people in the United States have diabetes and more than 90% of the cases diagnosed are among overweight or obese adults. Other risk factors for developing diabetes include inactivity, family history, gestational diabetes, and ethnicity; African, Latino, Native Americans Asian and some of Pacific Island ancestry.

Adults with diabetes are two to four times more likely to die of heart disease or stroke, and two-thirds have high blood pressure and mild to severe forms of nervous system damage, which is a major contributor to limb amputations. Furthermore, diabetes is the leading cause of blindness in adults between the ages twenty to seventy-five, with 24,000 new cases of blindness annually. The death rate in infants born to women with diabetes is triple that of newborns born to healthy mothers. During the last ten years, the incidence of diabetes tripled for ages eighteen and under. 123,000 diagnosed cases are under the age of twenty. Diet and exercise has tremendous implications in the prevention of diabetes, heart disease and stroke.

HYPERTENSION

Hypertension is a condition commonly known as high blood pressure, which affects 60 million Americans, and the leading cause of heart disease, stroke and kidney failure. There are two measurements important in hypertension: the systolic pressure, when the heart beats; and, the diastolic pressure, when the heart rests. A blood pressure value of 120/80 is considered optimal, and a reading of 130/85 is accepted as normal. Everyone experiences changes of blood pressure on occasion. The hypertension begins when the blood pressure goes up and stays up. There are two types of hypertension: primary hypertension, and secondary hypertension. In primary hypertension, the body is unable to control blood pressure and the condition is genetically inherited. Secondary hypertension results from hormonal drug therapy, decongestants, eating habits, stress and smoking. Although there is no known cure for hypertension, the condition can be managed by eating healthy, losing the extra weight, exercising regularly and not smoking.

RECENT CHANGES IN THE FOOD SUPPLY, AND AMERICAN PREFERENCES

The food supply is very different today than it was during the 1950's. First of all, the meats we consume contain 30% more fat compared to the 3% fat in the meats consumed by our ancestors. In the past, animals raised for food were shepherded; today, animals are raised in captivity and therefore, they develop more fat. In addition, science and technology have improved the foods for longer shelf life, fortification of needed nutrients, as well as taste and texture. The result is plenty of food to choose from that is appealing and tasteful, but contains more fat, sugar and salt. Furthermore, the shopping habits of the American consumer reveal that food choices are influenced first by personal taste, followed by cost, cultural preference, lifestyles, social and emotional comfort, body image and nutrition. Therefore, when it comes to choosing food, most of us consider taste and cost first and nutrition last.

The major issue of weight is no longer just about looking good. **It is also about being healthy**. *Americans want to be healthy, improve their physical performance and look good.* <u>*If that is true, why are so many of us overweight, when there is so much information on nutrition and health available?*</u>

In the last ten years, Americans have undergone tremendous lifestyle changes, which are responsible for the overall gain in body fat. The major factors that have contributed to being overweight or obese are:

- We eat huge food portions!
- Increased efficiency in food preparation
- We no longer work to prepare the food.
- We spend half of our food money on already prepared and pre-packaged food products that are high in fat and calories.
- Inactivity. We have become sedentary in recent years.
- We eat in restaurants often.

Most family style restaurants today advertise all you-can-eat buffets or offer extra large portion sizes to entice people to buy more food for less money; but we are not saving money, we are storing more fat. When we eat an appetizer, soup, salad, main entrée and dessert, we have most likely consumed over three thousand calories for just one meal. We consume more food than any other nation in the world!

Another reason contributing to the problem of weight gain is the amount of diet aids and weight loss diets available, claiming easy solutions to losing weight quickly. Every year, magazine covers advertise new approaches to lose weight fast for the holidays, the summer and every occasion that one can imagine. Let's not forget the abundance of advertisements that claim exercise in a bottle, and the pill that would trap all the fat, carbohydrates and sugar you can eat. Quick answers to our weight problems, including diets that specify only certain foods and omit others, <u>are not healthy.</u> Quick answers to losing weight are only traps into a roller-coaster ride, losing and gaining weight, with each attempt ending in another failure, and the next attempt becoming even more difficult. There are many healers ready to offer quick solutions for losing weight by proposing different diets, including high protein and fat.

Many people believe that high protein diets make you thin and promote more muscle, and that carbohydrates will promote the development of fat. <u>Not true.</u> Yes, we do need protein, but only a small amount. <u>Quick weight loss has very limited possibilities</u>. Even if we stop eating entirely, the most we can lose is half a pound a day (the amount of fat used will be equaled to the energy burned while fasting). Carbohydrates are a clean fuel source for the body; their waste products are carbon dioxide and water and they provide the most efficient fuel for energy needed for brain, heart and lung function. When proteins and fats become the main source of energy, the body has to *convert the protein to carbohydrates and use fats for energy through a more complex chemical reaction, and therefore the kidneys use more water to filter out all the impurities through the urine. This process results in dehydration and weight loss due to water loss, not fat loss.* <u>*High protein diets promote dehydration not weight loss.*</u> *In addition, high protein diets cause a dangerous condition called "ketosis," which is one of the conditions that makes diabetics ill, due to an inability to use carbohydrates efficiently.*

Another health risk with high protein diets (from animal sources) is the amount of fat they contain, even when the meat consumed is lean. In addition to dehydration and ketosis, a diet consisting mostly of animal protein causes nutrient deficiencies and heart disease. The Council on Foods and Nutrition has issued warning statements on "high protein diets" cautioning people with heart disease, kidney problems, high blood pressure, and pregnant women. This alone should be a clue that a high protein diet from animal sources is not healthy, and the quick weight loss is largely due to dehydration; once a normal eating pattern is resumed, the weight is quickly regained.

We spend thirty-five billion dollars every year on weight loss programs to no avail. Most Americans diet on and off, 92% report purchasing reduced calorie products, and only a small fraction of the population follow the established guidelines for diet and exercise recommended by the experts. We eat too many calories, too much fat and sugar, not enough vegetables and fruit, not enough fiber-rich foods or foods rich in calcium, and most of us practice a sedentary life style.

Research shows that the people who restrict their food intake severely find themselves binging (eating too much food at one time) on high fat and high calorie foods, consuming a lot more food than they would have eaten if they had simply eaten regularly. If binging on food is repeated often, it is considered to be a disorder, occurring mostly in women, and can lead to bulimia, anorexia, and obesity promoted by a stress response to severe restriction of food intake.

CURRENT LIFESTYLE TRENDS

An equally important reason for the high incidence of obesity is that we are simply inactive. Technology has made our lives easier. Adults and children are less active today than even a decade or two ago. It is not bad enough that we drive instead of walking to the grocery store, the bakery, the cleaners, the pharmacy or the bank. We no longer know nor recognize these proprietors, as we never see them because technology enables us to reduce our activity and isolate ourselves socially.

We can order anything we need via the Internet or telephone and have it delivered to our door. Many of us do our shopping for clothes, household items and even for large items such as a car or a home through the Internet. It takes a lot of calories to walk around the mall to find the items you want. We hire gardeners to do simple garden tasks that burn considerable calories, and we take our car to the car wash and pay other people to use their energy, as we stand and watch.

We spend a lot of time on the Internet playing games, e-mailing or using the computer for a home-based business, requiring little energy. In addition, our children pick up our bad habits.

SNACKING

Snacking is eating or drinking any amount of food outside the structure of mealtime; breakfast, lunch and dinner. Supermarkets and convenient store aisles are filled with chips, soda, candy and other snack foods high in fat, sugar and salt. In 1998 the Snack Foods Association reported that Americans spent over 70 billion dollars on snack food products, not counting fruits, vegetables, or beverages. In addition, we consumed 5.9 billion pounds of salted snack foods, with the average adult consuming over 500 calories per day from high fat and calorie snack foods. As with other things, Americans are also teaching the rest of the world to follow in their footsteps. The USDA reported that snack food exports have increased by 45% since 1992 in countries like Canada, Mexico, Japan, China, Australia, and Western European countries.

The Journal of the American Dietetic Association in 1994 stated that the U.S. adult population snacks two to three times per day. Among children, snacks were consumed three to four times a day and most people underestimated the amount of food they ate in a given day. Twenty years ago, the American teenager consumed twice the amount of milk as soda pop. Today, twenty percent of the total intake of calories comes from soft drinks, and even though we have decreased the consumption of fat in recent years, we are still consuming too much. The daily consumption of fat recommended by the USDA is 30% or lower of the total calories: this percentage includes the fat that is consumed when eating meat or dairy products, butter on the bread and salad dressing.

Sodium consumption is also on the increase. The recommended amount is 2,400 mgs per day, but we consume twice this amount. Most processed foods contain large amounts of salt, which can contribute to problems with high blood pressure, calcium leaching from the bones, and additional problems in people who are salt sensitive. The body retains water when we are dehydrated; excess salt can be excreted by drinking water to carry the salt out. Snacking can be healthy by eating five small and nutritious meals to keep the blood sugar stable, which will ultimately contribute to weight loss.

OSTEOPOROSIS

Another health problem we are facing today is a disease called osteoporosis, and it is not a result of obesity; it is the result of poor eating habits and an unbalanced diet. Osteoporosis is the reduction of bone tissue caused by calcium deficiency and is responsible for approximately 1.5 million bone fractures every year. Of the people with bone fractures, twenty percent die within a year and *half of those who survive need assistance for the remainder of their life. This accounts for billions in health care and other related costs annually. These costs come out of everyone's pocket; as the demand for care increases, the cost of insurance premiums also increases, leaving many people unable to afford insurance. Unless we do something about our current eating habits and lifestyle, and treat the problem with some urgency as a country, our lives will be further threatened and health care costs will continue to increase.*

RISK FACTORS FOR OSTEOPOROSIS

Family history

Low calcium intake throughout life

Sedentary lifestyle

Cigarette smoking

Excessive alcohol consumption

Thin body type

Women with no pregnancies

The Importance of Calcium

Calcium is a very small organic matter found in abundance in marble, limestone, eggshells and pearls. It is an essential dietary mineral with a profound effect on the human body. It strengthens our skeletal structure, enables the body to support our weight when we stand, stops bleeding, helps our muscles contract when we move, and helps regulate blood pressure in addition to other important functions. Recent research on the needs of calcium throughout life has prompted the re-evaluation of the recommended daily requirements. Findings also reveal that most of us fail to meet the requirement for calcium, despite the abundance of information on calcium and its association to bone disease. Another factor that contributes to the problem is that most people are unaware of the importance of calcium in the diet.

CALCIUM BALANCE

Calcium balance is difficult to achieve because the amount of calcium absorbed by the body with normal intake of food is between 25% and 30%. In addition, some dietary components can form insoluble products in the intestine that prevent calcium from being absorbed, and calcium is therefore lost in the urine or feces. Additional losses of calcium are shed through the skin, hair and nails. Ninety-nine percent of the body's calcium is in bone and teeth; the other one percent is in body fluids helping to regulate nerve transmission and muscle contraction, clotting of blood, and collagen maintenance, which is important in holding cells together. The daily requirement for calcium is determined by what is needed to maintain and support growth of the skeleton, as well as to replace what is lost through metabolic processes. Our body is in constant state of bone formation and dissolution, which requires calcium replacement.

Calcium requirements vary according to age and gender. Optimal calcium balance is achieved when the intake of calcium is enough to maximize peak adult bone mass and maintain adult bone mass, and to prevent bone loss later in life. However, calcium absorption decreases during the first decade of adulthood, while calcium deposition continues even after height has been achieved (linear bone growth stops by age twenty-two in males and age eighteen in females). Furthermore, maximum bone strength is not reached until age thirty for both males and females. During this decade, meeting calcium requirement is essential.

Calcium can be lost from the body due to excess consumption of certain dietary components. For example, excess sodium increases calcium losses by pulling the calcium with it in the urine. High amounts of protein, especially sulfur-containing amino acids, also have a negative effect on calcium retention by coupling with sulfates to pull calcium out with the urine. Additionally, foods containing oxalate prevent calcium from being absorbed, if consumed during the same meal. Oxalate is a salt of oxalic acid found in spinach, rhubarb, beet leaves and roots, lettuce, peanuts, snap beans, carrots, cocoa products and tea. Absorption or excretion problems associated with calcium and other foods can be avoided by planning your meals wisely. It is not that difficult; a dairy snack such as one cup of milk, one ounce of cheese or a cup of yogurt twice a day can provide over 500 milligrams of calcium.

Bone losses occur rapidly in women during the first three years of menopause, due to a sharp decline of estrogen. Adequate intake of calcium throughout life, vitamin D and weight bearing exercises are effective in the fight against bone loss during menopause. Unfortunately, once the bone matrix has been lost there is very little we can do, in terms of therapeutic intervention, to restore bone mass back to normal. Currently, scientists are researching possibilities for bone replacement therapy. Recent studies on calcium supplements reveal that supplementation slows bone loss when dietary calcium is inadequate.

A woman's calcium needs are very important during pregnancy and lactation. In the womb, calcification for baby teeth begins during the fifth month of gestation, and is completed by the time the baby starts teething. If the mother does not consume enough calcium during pregnancy, the fetus will take what it needs to grow, thus leaving the mother with a deficit of calcium for her own needs. Furthermore, breast milk contains 280 mgs of calcium per liter; during lactation, the mother can loose up to one percent of bone mass for each month that she breastfeeds.

As for the infant, calcium needs are greater at infancy than any other period of life; low birth weight infants may have higher requirements for calcium. As a child grows, the calcium needs remain high in proportion to body size because calcification for the wisdom teeth begins around the age of nine, when linear growth of bones is high. Lengthening of bones takes place in spurts with the last and largest growth spurt during puberty. The retention of calcium however, decreases as the child grows.

The teenage years are critical for achieving optimal bone mass. Forty-five percent of the adult skeleton is developed during the teenage years, because of a three-fold increase in bone mass. During the first decade of adulthood calcium deposition continues even if adult height has been achieved, and calcium depletion and replacement is continual throughout life.

CALCIUM SUPPLEMENTATION

The average American consumes approximately 800 mgs of calcium per day, falling short 200-500 mgs depending on age and gender. As stated before, dietary calcium, healthy eating, and weight-bearing exercises are important to promote and maintain healthy bones. Calcium supplements can help, but should not be the primary source of calcium. Talk to your physician or registered dietitian for a dietary assessment. Supplements should only be taken when the dietary calcium is inadequate to meet an individual's requirements. Calcium supplements greater than 500 mgs may have side effects such as constipation, intestinal bloating and excess gas. Taking 500 mgs or less is more easily tolerated by the stomach and the intestinal system. Remember, supplements cannot replace food! Food sources of calcium contain other essential nutrients important in maintaining optimal health.

Recommendations For Choosing Calcium Supplements

Always read the label.

Choose supplements with a high percentage of calcium (40% or greater).

Ask the pharmacist for calcium supplements that can be easily dissolved and absorbed.

Choose supplements manufactured by a reputable company.

Make sure it has the USP sign stamped on the label. USP means that <u>the United States Pharmacopoeia has tested the product for potency, purity and dissolvability.</u>

Avoid natural sources of calcium (bone meal, dolomite and oyster shell). These sources may contain lead or other heavy metals.

Divide calcium doses throughout the day, taking the maximum dose of 500 mgs at one time with twelve ounces of water.

The best sources of calcium are dairy foods, due to their calcium content and our body's ability to absorb them.

THE BEST FOOD SOURCES OF CALCIUM

Food Source	Calcium (Mgs)
3 oz canned sardines	370
1 cup milk	297
2% milk fat	297
1 cup buttermilk	296
1 cup low-fat yogurt	294
12 oz Cappuccino	260
1 oz American cheese	230
1 cup cottage cheese	230
13-19 medium oysters	225
1 oz cheddar cheese	200
3 oz canned pink salmon	167
2 tablespoons grated Parmesan	170
1/3 cup almonds	130
½ cup steamed broccoli	135
½ cup turnip greens	125
½ cup soft-serve ice cream	115
½ cup steamed mustard greens	97
½ cup sautéed Chinese cabbage	90
½ cup ice cream	85
3 dried figs	80
8 pods okra	78
1 medium orange	50

CALCIUM REQUIREMENTS ACCORDING TO AGE

AGE GROUP	MGS CALCIUM
0-3	500 mgs
4-8	800 mgs
Males	
9-18	1300 mgs
19-50	1000 mgs
>50	1200 mgs
Females	
9-18	1000 mgs
19-50	1000 mgs
>50	1500 mgs
Pregnant or Lactating women	1500 mgs <u>Or</u> an additional serving from the dairy group per day.

Because it is difficult to achieve a positive calcium balance, many food products today are fortified with calcium. To help prevent osteoporosis and preserve bone strength it is important to consume adequate intake of calcium and Vitamin D throughout life, avoid smoking, reduce alcohol intake, and do bone-strengthening exercises every day.

Ways To Increase Consumption of Calcium

- Eat low-fat yogurt for breakfast or snack, with fresh fruit instead of pre-mixed.

- Add one ounce of low-fat grated cheese to your salad.

- Drink juice fortified with calcium.

- Make dips with cottage cheese or yogurt.

- Eat dark green and leafy vegetables every day.

- Eat dried beans or peas at least three times per week.

- Order a Cappuccino or Latte as your choice of coffee.

- Include low-fat hard cheese on your sandwich instead of mayonnaise.

- Consume orange juice and other foods that are fortified with calcium.

CHAPTER 2

CURRENT FOOD AND EXERCISE TRENDS AMONG OUR CHILDREN

The average American child spends five to six hours per day watching television and playing video games. It is no wonder the current statistics for obesity in children and adults are alarming. Television viewing and video games are the most prevalent sedentary behaviors contributing to the recent incidence of obesity among young children and teenagers in the United States. Television viewing is responsible not only for inactivity, but also for overeating. Eighty–five percent of all food advertisers promote high fat, high sugar and highly salted food products.

Schools are partly responsible for what our children eat, and some do not provide physical education or encourage every child to participate in sports as part of the curriculum. Fast foods on school campuses increased by 600% from 1991 to 1996 alone. Schools contract brand-name fast food companies to provide and serve lunch without any nutritional requirements imposed. I taught high school for seven years and watched teenagers eat their lunch. A typical school lunch is a greasy burger, fries and soft drink. And for dessert we offer them candy, ice cream, sweet rolls and more soft drinks. We have gone from 6.5 ounces soft drink servings during the early 1970's to 20 ounces today. Teenage boys drink an average of three 12-ounce cans of soft drinks per day and about 10% of them drink five cans per day.

Teenagers today receive mixed messages. On the one hand, they see magazine and television advertisements telling them to be thin, and on the other hand, they are receiving messages to eat more foods that are high in fat and calories with little nutritional value. When our children go to school, an institution that we tell them to respect, they should be provided with nutrition and fitness knowledge in word and practice. However, only a very small percentage of our children know the importance of good nutrition. Currently, the curriculum in schools is not designed to teach our children about the importance of good nutrition and exercise. Nutrition classes and physical education should be a requirement in every school, and for every child, and the lunch program should offer foods that taste good and are nutritionally adequate to meet our children's needs.

Children do not need to count calories, but they need nutrient dense foods from all the food groups and need to be physically active. In families where both parents work, children spend their time watching television, playing videogames and eating "empty calorie" foods. To make matters worse, some parents think if a child is overweight he or she must be adequately nourished. On the contrary, most overweight children are deficient in nutrients such as calcium, iron, folacin and zinc.

One of the more serious medical problems among children today is Type II diabetes, which two decades ago primarily occurred among overweight adults over forty years of age. Most of the children diagnosed with Type II diabetes are overweight. Research shows that children who eat at regular meal times with the family, tend to eat slowly, recognize when they are full and eat healthier than children who are unsupervised during meals. Parents are the most influential factor in their children's eating behavior before they reach puberty, and therefore, it is very important for them to model a healthy eating behavior. On the other hand, research on eating behaviors and food choices among teenagers, shows that they are influenced most by peers and the environment.

Just like adults, overweight children also suffer from negative self-image, depression, low self-esteem and social isolation. Even very young children express negative attitudes towards other children who are fat. Negative body image in children starts as early as six years of age, and a comprehensive evaluation for weight management is not complete unless the following factors are considered:

- *Evaluate the family system and how you communicate.*

- *How much your family members know about their risks and nutrition.*

- *Are there any self-esteem issues that need to be addressed?*

- *Is the family member depressed or having behavioral problems?*

- *Is physical fitness an important part of every day life to the family unit?*

Major factors contributing to childhood obesity are:

- *Limited opportunities for outdoor play.*
- *The issue of safety.*
- *Reduction in family size.*
- *The elimination of physical education in schools.*
- *Being driven to school.*
- *Increase in technology in the home.*

Inactivity and poor eating habits are major factors contributing to poor health in children. Very few of our children go outdoors to play or ride their bikes after school, and most children today are playing computer games or watching television. If we hypothetically compare two children of the same weight and height and both eat the same amount of food every day, but one child plays two hours of soccer three times a week, and the other child plays computer games of the same amount of time, which of these two children is more likely to become obese? The obvious answer is the child playing the computer games. The child who plays soccer requires more calories, but he or she is also increasing the metabolic rate to burn more calories at rest, because this child has developed more muscle. More muscle mass naturally requires more calories for energy and therefore, the child who is active can eat more food. Keep in mind that muscle weighs more than fat; it is biologically more active and requires more calories for maintenance, and in addition, it promotes efficient use of energy. On the other hand, the child watching television is being sedentary and encouraged to eat more junk food promoted by advertisements.

Dietary management, physical activity and behavior modification are important steps in maintaining normal weight. Behavior modification may be necessary when a child uses food for comfort, or when television and video games take up the majority of the child's time.

HEALTHY FOOD HABITS FOR THE WHOLE FAMILY

Model good health habits for your children. They learn by example.

Choose foods that have variety and different texture every day.

Select foods with high water content and fiber, such as fresh fruits and vegetables.

Have fresh fruit available for snacking.

Cut fresh vegetables in small pieces for finger foods and store on a refrigerator shelf where small children can reach.

Make it a rule for your young children to eat fresh fruits and vegetables daily.

For a more satisfying snack, choose foods that contain protein, carbohydrates and some fat.

Choose cereals that contain less than 3 grams of sugar per serving and serve with low-fat milk.

Offer milk or water as the first options for a beverage.

BEHAVIOR MODIFICATION FOR YOUNG CHILDREN

Children should eat small frequent meals or snacks, starting with breakfast, and up to four times a day.

The whole family should eat together at least twice a day.

Take an active part in what your children eat and supervise their eating behavior.

Do not force your children to finish all their food.

Make sure that mealtime is socially and emotionally enjoyable.

Take your children food shopping, and let them choose some of the fresh vegetables and fruits; they will be more accepting in eating them.

Let your child help with cooking and emphasize the importance of good nutrition during this time.

Make an effort to prepare recipes that taste good.

All the family members should eat the same type of food at mealtime-only the portion sizes should vary.

Make older children responsible for preparing a healthy dinner at least once a week.

HEALTHY SNACKS FOR CHILDREN

Fresh fruit.

One stalk of celery with 1-tablespoon peanut butter spread.

One slice cheese with three wheat crackers.

½ cup cottage cheese served with ½ cup fresh fruit.

¼ cup dried almonds, walnuts or peanuts.

Whole grain cereal served with fruit and low-fat milk.

A cold slice of boneless chicken or turkey on whole wheat bread served with sliced tomatoes and cucumbers.

1- cup plain yogurt served with fresh fruit slices.

1- cup milk served with 2 Graham crackers.

½ Tuna fish sandwich made with whole wheat bread.

Fresh raw vegetables (carrots, peppers, zucchini, cucumbers, broccoli and celery) sliced and served with ¼ cup yogurt dip (see recipe in the cookbook section).

Diet Recommendations For Children 2-12 Years of Age

1-2 Servings meat, poultry, eggs or nuts; two times a week.

2 Servings fish; three times a week.

2-4 Servings (¼) cooked legumes; beans, lentils or peas; at least twice a week.

2-3 Servings milk or milk substitute, such as yogurt and cheese.

4 Servings fruit, with at least one serving from citrus.

4 Servings from green, red, orange and yellow vegetables; with at least one serving from leafy vegetables.

2-4 Servings from bread, cereal, pasta or rice.

1-2 Tablespoons olive oil in cooked food or in a salad.

*See chapter five for serving sizes

Diet Recommendations For Teenagers

2 Servings from meat, chicken, eggs or nuts; two times a week.

3 Servings from fish, three times a week.

2 Servings legumes: beans, lentils and peas, two times a week.

4 Servings low fat milk or milk substitute (yogurt or cheese).

4 Servings fruit, with one of the four servings from citrus fruit or juice.

5-6 Servings from green, red, orange and yellow vegetables; with at least one of serving from leafy vegetables.

4-8 Servings bread, potatoes, cereal, pasta or rice.

2-4 Tablespoons olive oil in cooked food or in a salad.

*See chapter five for serving portions.

CHAPTER 3

OUR NUTRIENT REQUIREMENTS

ENERGY NEEDS

Millions of years ago the human metabolism evolved to store fuel derived from overeating as body fat to be used during periods of famine. Today our metabolism is essentially the same and while one-third of the world population is experiencing famine, we have too much to eat and we overindulge. The human body depends on calories from food sources to use for energy. However, calories consumed should equal calories used up for body maintenance and energy. Simply stated, if the calories consumed are more than the calories used for fuel daily, the body will maintain a "check and balance" system very much like the one used in banks for deposit and withdrawal. Over a period of time, if the excess in calories deposited is not used up or withdrawn, they will accumulate resulting in weight gain. Our body will store the excess calories consumed as body fat. When the body has accumulated 3,500 calories more than it needs for energy, over a month or just a few days, a pound of fat is added to body fat stores. The reverse will be true for losing a pound of weight when we consume 3,500 calories less than what the body requires. The total calories needed by the body every day are used to fuel metabolic function and the energy needed for daily life and exercise.

Metabolism is a biochemical reaction that occurs in the body's cells and is influenced by the level of activity, type of food, and the amount that we eat. Basal metabolism is a necessary process for the maintenance of life; the beating of the heart, inhaling oxygen and exhaling carbon dioxide, maintaining body temperature, brain and nerve function, and all other metabolic activities that take place in every cell of our bodies. Thus, the Basal Metabolic Rate (BMR) is the minimum energy needed by the body before any type of physical activity is performed. A person's metabolism is influenced by age, gender, size and physical condition, and partly genetics. We all know at least one or two people who can eat anything they want, be completely inactive and still not gain a pound. These people have a higher metabolic rate or energy expenditure than the average person and need more calories to fuel their body. People who have a low metabolic rate gain weight easier because their body needs fewer calories for maintenance.

Furthermore, the younger we are the more calories we need to sustain life, due to the increased activity within the cells. When we are young our cells undergo division and replacement rapidly, especially during growth spurts. Once adult height has been reached, after the age of twenty, the metabolic rate decreases 5% with every decade. Another factor influencing the metabolic rate is the amount of lean tissue mass. Muscle tissue is active even when a person is at rest; males have a much higher metabolic rate than females who normally have less muscle and more fat tissue. Compared to muscle tissue, fat tissue is inactive and needs fewer calories for maintenance. Fasting and low-calorie diets lower the basal metabolic rate (BMR), partly due to loss of lean tissue and decreased metabolic functions. A protective mechanism in the body conserves energy during a time when the body perceives an energy shortage, such as fasting or when the body is deprived of food.

Epinephrine is a hormone secreted by the adrenal glands into the blood stream, when a person is excited, and temporarily increases the BMR. But, the most effective way to raise the basal metabolic rate is with exercises such as jogging or hiking. The basal metabolic rate is high during exercise and remains high even after the activity is completed, which is the reason why exercise is such an important part of weight management. People who want to maximize fat loss through exercise should consider choosing moderate level activities, such as walking and bicycling, to help maximum utilization of body fat. Exercise will be discussed at a later chapter.

A balanced diet can easily be achieved by choosing nutrient dense foods from all the food groups and by controlling the amount you eat. A nutrient is a substance essential to human development, growth and maintenance. Food from different food groups is made up of nutrients such as proteins, carbohydrates and fats. These nutrients contain calories, as well as vitamins and minerals, and other components essential for life. Calories consumed from food that do not contain nutrients are called "empty calories" and should be consumed sparingly. Alcoholic beverages, soft drinks and candy are good examples of empty calorie food products. On the other hand, foods that are rich in nutrients, but relatively low in calories are considered to be "nutrient dense," and should make up the largest portion of the daily food consumption. These foods come from meat, fish, legumes, dairy products, vegetables, fruits, whole grain products and olive oil. Prepared food products, such as canned or processed, are not the best sources of nutrients because they contain preservatives, too much sodium and saturated fat, and other additives that enhance palatability, texture and appearance.

CARBOHYDRATES AND PROTEIN

Carbohydrates *are synthesized in green leaves of plants from carbon dioxide and water, using the energy of sunlight. Carbohydrates are primarily found in plant food sources and are the body's most efficient fuel source. Other less efficient fuel sources are protein, fat and alcohol. Complex carbohydrates are starch and fiber with cellulose being the fiber part of the plant. On the other hand, simple carbohydrates are derived from refined sugars, such as cane sugar, candy, cakes and other pastries. Carbohydrates from food are converted to glucose, the form of energy used by the cells for various functions. If the blood delivers more glucose than the cells need, the muscles and* *liver take up the excess and store it in the liver as glycogen. If there is a severe carbohydrate deficit, as in fasting, the body depends on the protein to make glucose. When protein is used to make glucose for energy, it is taken from muscle and blood protein, which prevents it from performing its primary functions. Protein is essential to important biochemical functions necessary to maintain good health and should not be used as an energy source. Furthermore, protein is not an efficient energy source; high amounts in the diet or when muscle protein is used for energy, results in dehydration causing the kidneys to work harder in removing protein byproducts. Carbohydrates, the best source of energy for the human body, must always be available to spare the protein for other biological functions.*

When blood glucose is too high, the pancreas reacts by releasing insulin to take glucose from the blood to the cells. The liver and muscles store a small portion as glycogen for later use, but are only able to store enough for a half day. The blood glucose levels quickly come down as the body stores the excess. On the other hand, when the glucose in the blood gets too low, the hormone epinephrine reacts by releasing glucose derived from liver glycogen.

When we eat a high concentrated sugar food like a candy bar, the blood glucose level will rise very quickly and the pancreas will respond immediately by secreting large amounts of insulin. Then, as the intake of sugar stops, the blood glucose level will drop drastically to below normal levels. But if we eat a complex-carbohydrate snack, like wheat toast and a piece of cheese, the delivery of glucose to the blood will take longer and the insulin response will be smaller, and it will result in healthy blood glucose levels. The fat in the cheese will slow down the digestion of carbohydrates and the protein will provide some amino acids, making more glucose available when needed.

When glycogen stores are depleted and blood glucose level is very low, and we still continue to deprive our body of food, the body will adjust by going into fasting mode. During this stage, the body breaks down muscle protein to provide glucose for the brain and uses body fat to fuel the remaining body cells. When this happens, the person will experience symptoms of hypoglycemia (anxiety, hunger and dizziness). The muscles become weak and trembling, and the heartbeat races in a struggle to provide more fuel to the brain. This is a signal that the body is experiencing an energy imbalance, and it may be dangerous.

As previously mentioned, glucose is essential to the functioning of every cell in the body, especially the nervous system. The body depends on plant foods for its source of energy; leaves, stems, roots, tubers, fruits, blossoms and seeds. Stems and leaves provide cellulose (fiber), are not high in calories and are not good as an energy source. Legumes and whole grain cereal (wheat, rice, oats, barley and corn) are very important to our diet because they provide the starch needed for energy, as well as vitamins and minerals. The problem is that in the last twenty years, we have been eating too many carbohydrates. We were told that carbohydrates were good and we decided that more was even better, thus eating large portions of bread with butter and pasta soaked in heavy cream sauces, and consuming large numbers of calories from saturated fat in addition to the carbohydrates. High carbohydrate diets are good for people who are very active, but for the average person who does most of their work sitting, it is overwhelmingly too much. Moderation applies to most things in life. If we eat too much from any one type of food, we will not be able to get the nutrients we need from other foods without overeating. Therefore, it becomes essential to plan a balanced diet and eat small portions.

<u>One gram of carbohydrates provides 4 calories</u>

Protein *is made of carbon, hydrogen and oxygen, and some proteins contain sulfur; all are linked into amino acid chains required by all body tissues for new growth and replacement of worn-out cells. Protein is necessary for the production of red blood cells, enzymes and hormones, to help transport fats and other nutrients, in maintaining tissue fluid balance, and in providing energy when all other sources of energy have been exhausted. Protein sources include eggs, seafood, red meat, poultry, dairy, legumes and nuts; they are an essential dietary component and should be consumed daily, but mostly from foods that are low in saturated fat.*

<u>One gram of protein provides 4 calories</u>

FATS

Fats are an essential part of the diet; they provide important fatty acids needed for metabolic body functions, and in the transportation and absorption of fat-soluble vitamins. The important question is, what type of fat do we need to consume and how much?

Saturated *fats are those found in many animal and some vegetable products. These fats are easily identifiable because they usually harden at room temperature. Foods high in saturated fats include beef, veal, lamb, pork, butter, cream, soft cheeses, whole milk products, cocoa butter, coconut oil and palm oil. Over-eating on foods containing saturated fat increases the level of cholesterol in the blood.*

Polyunsaturated *fats are found in vegetable oils: safflower, sunflower, sesame seed, corn, soybean and cottonseed oils. These fats are liquid in room temperature, and in moderate amounts, they are beneficial to health. In addition,* ***Omega-3*** *fatty acids are polyunsaturated fats found in the oils of fish and shellfish, and can actually lower the levels of triglycerides and LDL levels (the bad cholesterol) in the blood, helping to fight against heart disease. In addition, Omega-3 helps to alleviate other disease such as arthritis, migraines and certain types of tumors.*
Triglycerides are fats made by the body from the foods we eat; they circulate in the blood and are stored as body fat. High levels of triglycerides in

the blood, causes an accumulation of plaque in the artery walls, which leads to heart disease.

Monounsaturated fats are also liquid at room temperature and come from vegetable oils, such as olive oil and canola. These monounsaturated fats are very important because they help lower the bad cholesterol [LDL] and protect the good cholesterol [HDL] thus, helping to reduce the risk of heart disease. In contrast to the polyunsaturated fats, monounsaturated fats are resistant to oxidation and maintain their healthy properties even during heating. The benefits of olive oil in the human diet have been well documented and proven for many years among the Mediterranean countries, especially the island of Crete, in Greece, where olive oil is the primary fat in the diet. This will be discussed in more detail in chapters four and five.

<u>One gram of fat provides 9 calories</u>

VITAMINS

Vitamin A is a fat-soluble vitamin and a powerful antioxidant essential to building healthy cells. It helps promote healthy vision, the development of bones, and protects against infection and dry skin. Beta-carotene is the best food source for vitamin A, found in dark leafy greens, and orange, red, and yellow vegetables and fruits. Foods rich in vitamin A also include fish, dairy products and liver.

The **B vitamins** are all water-soluble and play a critical roll in cell growth, protect against infections, promote healthy brain and nerve functioning, and help prevent anemia.

Niacin (B3) helps convert food to energy, aids in digestion, promotes a normal appetite and healthy nerve function. The best sources for niacin are enriched fortified grain products, legumes, organ meats, peanut butter, poultry and fish.

Pyridoxine (B6) plays a vital role in transporting amino acids in protein metabolism, promoting the use of protein in making and repairing body cells, and fighting against infection. The best food sources for B6 are meats, liver, vegetables and whole grain.

Thiamin is important in carbohydrate metabolism and the utilization of glucose by the cells, it promotes proper functioning of muscles and nerves, and promotes a healthy heartbeat. The best sources of thiamin are port, liver, yeast, legumes, and green vegetables.

Cobalamin (B12) helps synthesize red blood cells and build the genetic material needed by the cells, helps the body use fatty acids and amino acids and may have a protective effect against memory loss. The best food sources for B12 are poultry, beef, fish, seafood, eggs, and low-fat dairy products.

Folic Acid prevents certain defects of the fetus during pregnancy. It helps construct the DNA and RNA in the regeneration of new cells that have protective properties to help fight against heart disease. The best food sources for folic acid are leafy greens, legumes, orange juice and wheat germ.

Riboflavin is important in breakdown of protein and fatty acids to produce energy, to transfer energy between compounds, and is indispensable to the release of energy from food. The best source of riboflavin is milk, followed by meat, liver, eggs, leafy greens and whole grains.

Vitamin C is water-soluble and it has antioxidant properties, which are important in healing wounds. Vitamin C helps promote healthy skin by building the cell walls, and by manufacturing collagen and strong connective tissue. Collagen is essential for strong ligaments, tendons, skin, blood vessels and bones. Vitamin C also boosts the formation of red blood cells by facilitating iron distribution and absorption, and acts as a barrier against harmful toxins by building resistance against allergies, viruses and infections. The amount of vitamin C consumed by Americans has dropped by 20% in the last thirty years. Recent research shows that low intake of vitamin C can lead to fatigue and listlessness. The best food sources for vitamin C are citrus fruits, citrus juices, tomatoes, broccoli, leafy vegetables, peppers and strawberries.

Vitamin D is a fat-soluble vitamin that increases the body's ability to absorb calcium. In addition to promoting strong teeth, vitamin D plays a critical role in developing and maintaining strong bones. The human body is able to produce its own vitamin

D when exposed to sunlight. The best food sources for vitamin D are milk, eggs, liver and fish.

Vitamin E *is a fat-soluble vitamin and powerful antioxidant. It protects the cells from damage and breakdown by guarding against destruction of other nutrients, and eliminating free radicals; it promotes healthy blood and the formation of hormones; it keeps metabolism in balance by conserving the body's supply of oxygen, thereby, strengthening the respiratory and immune system to guard against disease. The best food sources for vitamin E are whole grain breads, cereals, peanuts, walnuts, soybeans, bran, wheat germ, wheat germ oil and avocado.*

Vitamin K *is a fat-soluble vitamin necessary for the clotting process within the blood cells. Vitamin K can be synthesized in the lower part of the intestines, but absorption takes place in the upper portion of the intestinal tract. The best sources of vitamin K are liver, leafy greens, broccoli, cauliflower, and garbanzo beans.*

MINERALS & TRACE ELEMENTS

The term **"mineral"** *refers to substances derived from the water and earth. Minerals are absorbed from the earth by plants. The animals that we eat as a food source also eat these plants. Therefore, plant and animal food products are a good source of minerals. The following minerals are essential to good health:*

Calcium and phosphorous are required by every cell in the body especially teeth, bones, heart and nerves. Calcium is discussed in greater detail in chapter one.

Phosphorous helps transport lipids in the blood and is an essential mineral for all cell growth. 85% percent of phosphorous is found coupled with calcium as bone crystals; as calcium phosphate, it gives strength and rigidity to bones and teeth. Phosphorous is found in most foods containing calcium and protein.

Iron is important for the formation of healthy red blood cells and necessary for the body's ability to utilize oxygen. The proteins in red blood depend on iron to help carry the oxygen to the cells. Iron deficiency anemia can result from many illnesses, but it can also occur if a person's diet is low in iron. A common symptom of anemia is a continuous feeling of tiredness. Even a balanced diet is not enough for some people because the body only absorbs 10-30% of the iron. Supplements arc usually recommended for menstruating, pregnant and lactating women and for children. The best food sources of iron are oysters, beef liver, red lean beef and veal, avocados, dried apricots, prunes and enriched bran cereal.

Zinc helps to heal wounds, promotes healthy taste buds, and is essential to protein metabolism. Oysters are the best food sources for zinc; other good sources are herring, egg yolks, beef, liver, legumes, milk and yogurt.

Selenium *has antioxidant properties powerful enough to be a substitute for vitamin E in fighting against the risk of many diseases. The best food sources for selenium are poultry, seafood, garlic, broccoli, tomatoes, onions, nuts, mushrooms and whole grain bread and cereal.*

Iodine *is essential for the formation of the thyroid hormone that regulates the body's metabolism. The thyroid hormone levels determine the rate that the body responds to the metabolism of energy, by controlling the rate of oxygen used by the cells as energy is released. Iodine is found in seafood products and purified sodium chloride, as in iodized table salt (sea salt loses its iodine content during the drying process).*

Magnesium *helps form the protein mechanism that is used to form energy when glucose stores are depleted. It also helps to relax the muscles after contraction and promote healthy tooth enamel. The best food sources of magnesium are animal food products, green leafy vegetables, nuts, oysters and scallops. Deficiencies are rare unless the person has experienced severe vomiting and diarrhea, or alcoholism.*

Potassium, *sodium and calcium, help promote a healthy heart rhythm; they are essential for nerve conduction and impulse, muscle contraction and water balance. Extreme dehydration can cause potassium deficiency, which results in muscle weakness.*

Sodium is important for proper functioning of the body, but taken in excess, it can be harmful. Excess sodium is filtered from the blood by the kidneys into the urine. If the body is deficient of sodium, the kidneys conserve it and send it back to the blood stream. This happens when the body is in starvation from lack of food or during exercise when heavy sweating takes place. Most foods contain sodium, except fruits.

Cobalt. Coupled with B12, cobalt is essential in the production of red blood cells. Cobalt is found mostly in animal products and in small amounts in green leafy vegetables.

Copper is important in the formation of red blood cells and the release of energy. It also helps the formation of collagen and in maintaining a protective shield around nerve fibers. The best food sources for copper are grains, shellfish, organ meats, legumes, dried and fresh fruits, and most vegetables.

Chromium is an essential element needed to metabolize glucose in association with insulin; it facilitates the use of glucose to produce energy. Deficiency of chromium impairs the effectiveness of the hormone insulin, which regulates glucose. Low levels of chromium in the human tissue have been linked to adult-onset diabetes and impaired growth in children.

Fluoride is essential in building and maintaining strong teeth, and builds strong bones that resist degeneration and osteoporosis. The best source of fluoride is water.

PHYTOCHEMICALS & ANTIOXIDANTS

Phytochemicals are natural compounds found in plant food sources; they help protect against diseases, especially heart disease and cancer.

Antioxidants are substances found in fresh foods that destroy harmful microorganisms (free radicals) entering the human body. The antioxidant action changes the free radicals into stable oxygen molecules by blocking their attack to the cell. Antioxidants help elevate high-density lipoproteins (HDL), which are valuable in the regulation of fats in the bloodstream and for protecting the artery walls from developing plaques. Vitamins C, E, A, selenium and chromium, olive oil, fruits and vegetables, onions and garlic contain antioxidants that have been proven to fight against cholesterol and the buildup of plaque in the arterial walls.

SUPPLEMENTS

If you decide to take a vitamin supplement, look for a reputable brand that has been around for a few years and choose a supplement that contains only one hundred percent of the Recommended Daily Value. Calcium supplement should be taken separately, as it is too bulky to be added with other vitamins in one tablet.

Americans spend more than three billion dollars annually on nutrition supplements. We are taking *too many supplements instead of eating healthy. Supplements cannot take the place of food! Our bodies need nutrients from food sources for growth and maintenance. All the nutrients we need are available in fresh food and are the best insurance we have for good health. Supplementation may be necessary for infants, pregnant women, nursing mothers and older adults, when individual requirements exceed what a normal diet can supply.*

We are all different in terms of weight and height, body frame size, age and activity level. These differences make it apparent that our diets should be tailored to individual energy needs and therefore, to different food amount requirements. A physically active man who stands 6' tall and weighs 180 pounds can consume twice as much food as compared to a woman who stands 5'2" and weighs 120 pounds, even if the woman is physically active.

SPECIAL NEEDS FOR OLDER ADULTS

The body's metabolic rate slows down as we age. We need less food to fuel our daily requirements. A lower metabolic rate requires fewer calories for energy; therefore, as we age, the requirement for calories decreases, but the need for more nutrients increases. Older adults should select low-calorie nutrient dense foods to prevent consuming too many calories, which results in weight gain. If we decrease our calories by 5% for every decade after the age of twenty, by the time we reach sixty years of age we need to eat 20% less calories per day. This makes exercise an essential part of daily life in order to stimulate the metabolic rate and burn more calories for fuel.

Research shows that older adults tend to eat very little meat, milk, fruits, vegetables and whole grain products; thus, they are deficient of important vitamins including protein, iron, zinc and calcium, and contributing to the mental confusion that is often experienced by older adults. Furthermore, they are also deficient in vitamins A, C and E, which are important in fighting against many diseases and protect against aging. Finally, as discussed in chapter one, calcium intake begins at infancy and must be maintained throughout life. Once bone matrix has been lost, it is not easy to replace it. Adequately nourishing your body with calcium and regular exercise can help prevent further bone loss. On the other hand, anemia from lack of iron in the diet can be the cause of fatigue and apathy, and prevents older adults from engaging in outdoor activities.

Fiber *consumption is important for everyone, but becomes more important with advanced age. Whole grain cereals, fruits and vegetables eaten daily will help keep the muscles of the intestinal track working. Fiber also helps bind cholesterol in the intestines to carry it out of the body. Many older adults also suffer from high blood pressure and need to reduce salt intake, which promotes retention of body fluids and contributes to further increase in blood pressure. Consuming lean meat and poultry, more fish, fresh vegetables and fruits,* low-fat dairy products, and small portions of whole grains and legumes will provide the extra nutrients needed during our later years. We should also avoid eating processed foods, and daily walks can help improve circulation and promote bone health.

NOURISH THE SKIN FROM WITH-IN

Aging is an inevitable process of life that everyone will experience. As we age our skin becomes dry, wrinkled and saggy as the muscles become soft and weak. In addition, our sense of taste and smell decreases and we find it difficult to breathe with the slightest climb of stairs. However, <u>it is within our power to slowdown the process of aging.</u> Our skin cells reproduce every eight hours and over one thousand brain cells die every day, more in people who smoke. When we are young each cell self-produces through a process called "mitosis" or "doubling" by which thousands of cells die constantly and thousands are being reborn. These cells are biologically programmed to die after they have divided a specific number of times. When this biological process occurs, the clock starts ticking and the aging process begins. By our 30th birthday, every cell in our body begins to change. This change can be postponed, prolonging youthfulness for decades, by eating a healthy diet and exercising every day of your life. Damage in the DNA (deoxyribonucleic acid is the genetic material in living organisms located in the cell nucleus), is caused by forces within the cell, exposure to chemicals, and what we eat. When we eat empty calorie foods containing sugar, salt, saturated fat and preservatives, our cells are *assaulted, causing cellular damage, which confuses the internal clock resulting in the acceleration of the aging process. Signs of aging include rough-dry skin that is easily prone to infections and allergies, and is often caused by a vitamin deficiency. Foods rich in vitamins A, C, E and selenium can help alleviate the problem. We can protect ourselves from aging by living a healthy lifestyle.*

BEST SOURCES OF VITAMIN A AND THEIR APPROXIMATE VALUE

FOOD SOURCE	VITAMIN A IU
1 oz beef liver	15,000
½ cup dandelion greens	10,500
½ cup pumpkin	7,800
½ cup carrots	7,500
½ cup spinach	7,200
½ cup collard greens	5,100
½ cup winter squash	4,300
½ cup sweet potatoes	8,500
½ cup mustard greens	4,060
½ cup cantaloupe	6,500
½ cup broccoli	2,363
1 peach	1,300
½ cup cooked tomatoes	1,000
½ cup tomato juice	950
½ cup asparagus	600
1 egg	580
½ grapefruit	550
½ cup cooked peas	430
½ cup summer squash	400

RELIEF FROM ALLERGIES

Millions of people suffer from allergies. An allergy is an accumulation of waste products that enter the body through inhalation, swallowing, or by contact with the skin. Allergies can occur from pollen, dust, mold, feathers, wool dyes, chemicals, foods, medicines, herbs, insect stings and skin shed by animals. The reaction occurs after the substance has been absorbed into the bloodstream, which stimulates the white blood cells to produce antibodies. The antibodies react against the offending substance producing a reaction that may affect the digestive system, lungs, eyes or nose. Allergy reaction symptoms include itchy eyes and throat, sneezing, coughing, watery eyes, wheezing or difficulty in breathing. People who suffer from allergies often experience a constant feeling of fatigue and irritability.

Consume foods rich in vitamins A, C, E and Selenium every day; these vitamins will help protect the respiratory track from irritants by rebuilding the bronchial cells and tissues. Vitamin C foods can help regenerate the cell walls by making more collagen, which will act as a barrier against harmful substances. The pulpy portion of citrus fruits is rich with bioflavonoids, which help built immunity against allergies. Selenium, vitamin A and E rich foods protect the cell membrane from damage and promote a strong respiratory system.

Chapter 4

Balance Your Diet

As previously discussed, our weight problems today are largely due to prosperity, technological advances, over-consumption of high calorie foods, not enough variety in our diet and lack of exercise. Fortunately there are solutions to the problem, but it requires patience, planning and adherence. When discussing the problem of being overweight, only one thing is certain; prevention is much easier than treating the problem. We must now reverse our bad habits, become more active and make smart food choices.

It seems obvious, the only way to be lean and healthy is to eat a variety of foods mostly from fresh sources, eat smaller portions, be active every day and allow enough time to lose the excess fat. Practicing good eating habits and living an active lifestyle is the best way to stay slim long-term, and in the process feel and look our best. It is never too late to start on the road to good health. We have the power to change the present and the future. Support from loved ones is important, but ultimately, it is up to the person with the problem to make the final decisions. Healthy eating and exercise are essential for growth and repair throughout life, and affects our vitality and physical appearance. A well balanced diet and exercise plan leads to better health, builds stamina, and is the best guarantee for health and enjoyment in the later years.

It is not realistic to think that we will <u>never</u> eat cake, cookies, pastries, ice cream, or bypass the pastry shop for the rest of our life. <u>Moderation is the key to good health.</u> The amount of "empty calorie" foods we consume, and how often, is an important factor in maintaining a healthy weight. Indulging in a piece of cake once a week will not increase body fat; it is what else we do or don't do. We can have that piece of dessert we want, but only on occasion, not every day. Increasing the amount of exercise time an extra hour or two will make up for the calories in that piece of cheesecake we plan to eat Sunday afternoon with friends.

In the last fifty years research shows that the people in the island of Crete, Greece, have among the lowest incidence of heat disease. More recent studies on the eating habits of people among the Mediterranean countries and the U.S. show that the people in the island of Crete eat the healthiest; they eat four times more fruits and vegetables than other Mediterranean countries studied, and six times more than the U.S. In addition, they eat small amounts of red meat and chicken, one sixth the amount consumed in the U.S.

In Ancient Crete, meat was eaten only when an animal was sacrificed to the Gods, and later, meat was consumed only on religious holidays. The ancient diet consisted of legumes, vegetables, nuts, fish, olive oil, dairy, fruits and wine; not very different from the way they eat today. Today their diet consists mostly of fresh vegetables and legumes, fish, dairy, small amounts of red meat and chicken, whole grains, fresh fruits and a moderate amount of wine mostly consumed with dinner. Fresh fruit and nuts take the place of dessert after dinner or as a snack, and yogurt with nuts and a drizzle of honey is regularly consumed as dessert. Furthermore, extra virgin olive oil is the primary source of fat in the diet, making up more than 20% of the total calories. Concentrated sweets consumption is the exception, not the rule.

In addition to their good eating habits, most of the people walk an average of two to three miles every day. Walking is a part of daily life to run errands, shop, and for pleasure. Children still play outdoors after school, and one rarely sees an overweight child or teenager. As for older adults, most live vital and active lives, and most are able to take care of themselves during the later years. People in this island, as well as other Greek islands, rarely eat greasy fast foods and other unhealthy snack foods. In addition, only a small percentage of the population has a computer in the home. At least for now!

How To Start Living Healthier

Start by living a more active life and making a rule to eat mostly fresh foods, with limited consumption of precooked or prepackaged. Eat smaller portions from a variety of fresh foods, limiting the number of meals you eat away from home. When you do eat out, choose the most nutrient dense menu items and avoid ordering deep fry foods or foods with heavy sauces. Nutrient dense foods are those foods containing high proportion of nutrients to calorie content.

Always plan ahead to avoid being tempted to eat unhealthy snacks. The morning meal is the most important, because it will provide you with the energy needed to begin your day. If you skip the morning meal, you will feel tired or sluggish and have problems concentrating. Eating a healthy breakfast will energize you and prepare you to take on the challenges of the day. It does not mean that you need to cook breakfast; a slice of toast with an ounce of hard cheese and half of a banana is sufficient. If you normally exercise in the morning, make certain to eat at least twenty minutes prior to your exercise routine. The morning meal should be small and contain protein, carbohydrates and a small portion of fat. While the carbohydrates will provide fast energy, the protein is needed to repair muscle fibers and rebuild the immune system, and a small amount of fat is necessary to help metabolize important fat-soluble vitamins. Eat small, healthy snacks between meals to prevent extreme drops in blood sugar that result in fatigue, impatience and irritability.

Keep only nutritious snacks, water and 100% fruit juice at home or at the office. Try drinking water as often as possible and if you find it difficult, try drinking water with a straw. This may encourage drinking more water throughout the day. Eat fresh healthy foods and do not adhere to diets that only permit certain types of foods, unless advised by your doctor. Most people who are trying to follow a restricted diet to lose weight end up going from one diet to the next the rest of their lives and straining their heart in the process.

ANYTIME HEALTHY SNACKS

- *Half of a small bagel with a tablespoon of peanut butter.*
- *Half of a pita and one ounce hard cheese.*
- *A hardboiled egg, sliced tomato and one slice bread.*
- *1-ounce walnuts and dried fruit mix.*
- *1-cup low-fat yogurt and ½ cup fresh berries.*
- *8 ounces of 100% fruit juice.*
- *Half a sandwich made with 2-ounces lean meat, lettuce and tomato slices.*
- *A small fruit.*
- *A small salad made with mixed greens and vinegar and olive oil dressing.*
- *1-cup low-fat milk and half of a banana.*

Fifteen Steps For Optimal Health

- *Consume most of your calories from fresh fruits, vegetables, legumes, olive oil and whole grain products.*

- *Include low-fat dairy products such as yogurt, low-fat milk or cottage cheese with your meal or as a snack.*

- *Limit red meat and chicken consumption to two times a week, and eat nuts, legumes and fish more often.*

- *Limit the amount of sweets you consume to once a week or occasionally.*

- *Use extra virgin olive oil as salad dressing to prepare your food instead of butter or other saturated fats.*

- *Eat leafy vegetables and tomatoes often.*

- *Choose fruits that are low in sugar such as citrus, berries, plums and peaches.*

- *Avoid eating high sodium foods.*

- *Make regular exercise a daily routine.*

- *If you drink alcohol, do it in moderation!*

  One drink for women and older adults and two drinks for men.

- *Make a habit of drinking water throughout the day.*

- *Do not smoke or permit others to smoke around you.*

- *Drink coffee and tea in moderation to avoid dehydration.*

- *Do not combine medications, drugs, alcohol and herbal remedies without your doctor's advice.*

- *Take time out for relaxation, and sleep at least 7 hours every day.*

Foods That Fight Against Diseases & Aging

Almonds are rich in calcium, vitamin E, iron and protein. Most of the calories in almonds come from fat, but it is 90% unsaturated and provides the same health benefits to the heart as olive oil.

Asparagus contains asparagines, an antioxidant which helps the kidneys eliminate wastes by stimulating the metabolism.

Avocados contain a plant fat called beta-sitosterol and monounsaturated fats. Together, these fats help lower the bad cholesterol (LDL) circulating in the blood. Avocados also contain lutein, which has been found to shrink prostate cancer cells, helps protect the eyes from cataracts and prevents muscular degeneration.

Beets provide some iron, which promotes healthy red blood cells and eliminates wastes from the intestines.

Bran is an excellent source of fiber, which helps eliminate wastes from the colon and is effective in lowering cholesterol.

Broccoli is one of the first vegetables discovered to have properties that fight against cancer; it contains sulforaphane, which is an anti-cancerous substance that stimulates the body to produce its own antioxidant to fight against carcinogens. It also helps to prevent blindness by protecting the *retinal cells of the eye from damage. Cabbage and cauliflower also have anti-cancer properties.*

Cabbage *is rich in iron and sulfur. The antioxidant properties in cabbage eliminate fat deposits and harmful microorganisms from the intestines.*

Celery *contains high levels of calcium, and is a prime source of magnesium and iron, promoting healthy red blood cells and a strong immune system.*

Cucumber *is a metabolic stimulant and excellent diuretic, helping to remove accumulated fluids that destroy the body's cells; thus it is are considered as a cell cleanser.*

Eggplant *contains alkaline minerals with an antioxidant protection. Eggplant is low in calories and produces a feeling of fullness after eating a small portion, and helps to eliminate accumulated wastes from the colon.*

Fish *is one of the most healthy food sources, rich in protein, vitamins, minerals and Omega-3 fatty acids. One of the best ways to achieve a more healthy diet is to substitute fish for red meat. A three-ounce portion of cooked fish provides half of the protein your body needs each day to build and maintain cells. Fish protein is easily digested and utilized by our body. Most fish and other seafood products are rich in minerals, naturally present in seawater, such as iron, copper and calcium. Fish is also rich in iodine, potassium and fat-soluble vitamins A and D. In addition to the valuable* nutrients, fish is low in total calories and fat. A 3-ounce portion of fish contains between 85-150 calories. Mackerel, salmon and tuna are among the richest sources of Omega-3 fatty acids. A considerable amount of Omega-3 is found in Atlantic halibut, swordfish, bluefish and shellfish.

Legumes contain folate and fiber; help to improve blood vessel function, reduce blood clotting, lower cholesterol and protect against heart disease. Beans for example, are rich in folic acid (B vitamin), which is important in controlling the level of homocysteine in the body. Some scientists believe that high levels of homocysteine (an amino acid in the body) may be responsible for damaging the heart muscle prior to the damage done by high levels of the LDL cholesterol. Folic acid, B-12 and B-6 have shown to clean up the excess homocysteine from the body. Pinto beans, navy, and black-eyed peas are especially rich in folic acid.

Garlic should be used in cooking or consumed raw as often as possible. Garlic is well known and frequently used among Mediterranean countries. It is an excellent source of selenium, an antioxidant that slows the process of aging, and helps to protect the body from environmental pollution. It is especially helpful in the breakdown of free radicals found in fatty deposits. Selenium and vitamin E help protect against destruction of cell membrane and genetic coding. In addition, both help in stabilizing blood pressure and promoting a strong immune system. Garlic is beneficial in any form, fresh or powder.

Leafy greens include collard, kale, spinach, chard, mustard, dandelions and beet greens. Leafy greens contain chlorophyll, a compound that is broken down during digestion to produce another substance that fights against cancerous growths. Leafy greens are also rich in vitamin C and other compounds that help protect the body from breast cancer, and cancer of the uterus. Most leafy vegetables are easy to prepare and take less than five minutes to cook.

Nuts are an important source of protein, zinc, and unsaturated fat; necessary for the formation of collagen, which promotes healthy skin. All nut products contain a lot of calories and therefore should be consumed in moderation.

Oats are high in fiber and if consumed routinely, it reduces the bad cholesterol (LDL) in the blood, thereby reducing the risk of heart disease.

Olive oil. Studies on the benefits of olive oil consumption consistently reveal that it helps fight against heart disease, promotes fullness and thus prevents over-eating. More recent studies show that olive oil is not as easily stored in the body as adipose fat. For years we have been told that fat is bad for us, but this statement does not apply to olive oil, it is the saturated fat from animal sources, margarine and shortening that we must avoid. Extra virgin olive oil is the pure juice of the olives without any additives. It can be used to prepare foods in a variety of different cooking methods, including baking and frying, due to its ability to withstand high temperatures without altering its nutritional component. A small amount of olive oil adds flavor and taste, promotes satiety and good health.

Onions contain antioxidants that help prevent blood clots from forming and help promote healthy blood levels of cholesterol.

Oysters are one of the richest sources of zinc, essential to the production of anti-bodies that fight against bacterial and viral infections.

Parsley is an excellent source of many nutrients and antioxidant; they help to increase the metabolism of oxygen, destroy microorganisms that are harmful to cells, and help maintain the elasticity of blood vessels.

Peppers are a great source of vitamin C that promotes collagen formation and wound healing. One medium green pepper contains more vitamin C than an orange. Red peppers are an excellent source of vitamin A, which is considered a miracle antioxidant. Green, red and yellow peppers help prevent the destruction of human cells and help to maintain youthful skin. The hot peppers provide additional health benefits; they contain capsaicin, which is a potent antioxidant that helps destroy carcinogens before they can cause damage to cells. The hotter peppers contain more capsaicin.

Sunflower seeds are rich in protein and zinc, and help protect the body from developing cancerous cells.

Soy, *even in small amounts, can help reduce the bad cholesterol (LDL). Edamane, unshelled fresh soybeans, are a good source of soy and taste delicious when sautéed with a little olive oil.*

Sweet potatoes, carrots and cantaloupe *are an excellent source of beta-carotene, an antioxidant important in fighting against the breakdown of healthy cells.*

Vegetable oils *help protect the heart, liver and kidneys; they regulate the removal of wastes and provide a transportation system for essential fat-soluble vitamins A, E, D, and K.*

Tomatoes *are an excellent source of lycopene and vitamin C, both powerful antioxidants that help boost the body's metabolism and immune system. Lycopene is the substance responsible for the red pigment in tomatoes and helps to protect the body from certain types of cancer, especially cancers of the stomach, bladder and colon. Tomatoes also function as a diuretic by stimulating the kidneys to remove harmful substances that threaten health. Fresh tomatoes, tomato puree and crushed tomatoes are all rich in lycopene, but note that lycopene is absorbed more efficiently when cooked or eaten with a small amount of vegetable fat, such as olive oil or canola. A recent study, examining tomato consumption and lycopene content in breast milk, revealed a higher level of lycopene in the breast milk among mothers who consumed tomato sauce products regularly, even higher than those who consumed fresh tomatoes.*

Winter Squash, *butternut, turban, pumpkin and Hubbard are rich in beta-carotene, well known for its powerful anti-cancerous properties. Beta-carotene is converted to its active form of vitamin A by the body.*

Yogurt *is made from fermented milk and contains high amounts of calcium. If you cannot tolerate milk or other dairy products, try yogurt as another option; the lactobacillus, a bacteria in yogurt, reacts as an antioxidant in destroying harmful bacteria in the body and promotes digestion.*

FRUITS

Apples *contain pectin, a natural antioxidant, which stimulates metabolism to burn fuel; thereby, limiting the amount of fat deposited as adipose tissue. In addition, pectin is a water-soluble fiber that helps reduce the LDL cholesterol circulating in the blood that causes clogging of the arteries. Other fruits high in pectin are pears, prunes, apricots and bananas.*

Bananas *contain potassium, vitamin B6 and biotin; they nourish body cells to protect against destruction. Bananas also help in stabilizing blood sugar levels and promote a healthy heartbeat.*

Citrus. *The flavor and nutritional benefits of citrus fruits are highly accepted around the world, making them the ideal fruit for good health and longevity. It has been well documented that citrus fruits are rich in vitamin C, minerals and fiber,* *which are essential for growth and development. Research studies on the benefits of citrus fruits repeatedly show their extraordinary power to fight against cancer, heart disease and many other chronic diseases. Citrus fruits contain potassium, folate, calcium, thiamin, niacin, phosphorous, vitamin B6, magnesium, copper, riboflavin and phytochemicals. You should be aware however, that vitamin C can easily be destroyed by heat and oxygen. Heating during pasteurization of the ready to drink juices destroys the vitamin C content by 25%. The Vitamin C content of the premixed citrus juices drops by 45 milligrams per cup, to zero by the fourth week after opening the container, and should be consumed within a week after purchasing. In addition, recent research shows the frozen reconstituted citrus juices to contain more vitamin C than the pasteurized premixed; the oxygen in the air destroys vitamin C during production, handling and storing. All citrus fruits are low in calories: one medium orange contains about 80 calories, a grapefruit contains 90 calories, and one tangerine contains 40 calories. Furthermore, all citrus fruits are an important source of carbohydrates needed for energy balance and do not contain cholesterol or sodium.*

Anemia is a worldwide problem that has serious nutrient-related health problems, such as poor growth and impaired psychomotor development in children, reduced physical performance and decreased cognitive function. Consuming citrus fruits every day can help supply the body with enough folate for new red blood cell production, growth and maturation; all essential to preventing anemia and birth defects. New scientific evidence suggests that long-term consumption of citrus foods also decreases the risk of cataracts (eye disease), the formation of kidney stones, and promotes healthy cognitive function in older adults.

Cranberries are a natural diuretic helping to eliminate excess body fluids. As an antioxidant, it helps detoxify the body from free radicals and stimulate metabolism. Cranberries also contain compounds that prevent bacteria from attaching to the surface of the bladder, thus preventing urinary tract infections. Because cranberries taste tart, they are easier to consume as juice or as sauce.

Grapes are rich with flavonoids and antioxidants that help destroy cancer-causing substances, and prevent blood clots that can lead to heart attack.

Raspberries, blackberries and strawberries help protect against heart disease; their insoluble fiber from the seeds helps to breakdown carcinogens and speed up their passage through the intestinal track. One cup of blackberries has more fiber than any other fruit. Eating berries regularly can help reduce the risk of cancer and protect healthy cells from damage. Fruits with blue pigments, such as cherries and plums, provide additional benefits; they contain anthocyanins, strong antioxidants proven to be effective in destroying several types of cancers.

Recommended Food Plan For Adults

Vegetables
4-6 servings orange, yellow, red, and green color vegetables, with one serving from leafy greens.

Legumes
Two ½ cup servings cooked legumes: lentils, peas or beans, twice a week.

Fish & Nuts
Eat two servings of fish three times a week and one serving of nuts per week.

Fruits
2-4 Servings of fruit with at least 1 serving of fruit coming from fresh citrus.

Dairy
2-3 Servings of dairy foods, and choose low fat.

Bread & Cereal
4-8 Servings bread, cereal, pasta or rice.
> [4-servings for women
> 8-servings for men]

Meat
Two 3-ounce servings extra lean meat or poultry, only two times a week.

Fat
2-4 tablespoons of olive oil, per day.
> [2-3 tablespoons for women
> 3-4 tablespoons for men]

CRETE

"Out of the dark blue sea lies an island called Crete, a rich and lovely land washed by the waves on every side" –Homer

The island of Crete is renowned for being one of the most beautiful islands in the Mediterranean and for its cultural contributions to world civilization. Crete is credited with a tremendous wealth of historical events, achievements and traditions of distinctive character, and held in high standard within Greece and the world. Crete is located in the middle of the Mediterranean basin, with the Aegean Sea on its northern shores, centered between Europe, Asia and Africa. It is a mountainous island rising from the sea with three of its highest mountains rising 8,000 feet above sea level. Among these three mountains are green hills and valleys covered with vineyards, olive groves, orange groves and streams. The island is approximately 155 miles long from east to west and thirty-three miles at its widest point from north to south, with over 600 miles of coastline. The ideal geographical position of the island is responsible for its remarkably diverse landscape within a distance of just a few miles. Very few places compare to its diverse beauty. Crete has four seasons with a mild winter, when the snow covers only the peaks of the mountains. In the spring there is an abundant variety of wildflowers, a truly spectacular sight! Despite its mountainous landscape, Crete is self-sufficient. Its rich soil provides a huge variety of crops and agricultural products, and palm and banana trees flourish close to its warm sandy beaches.

CHAPTER 5

PORTION SIZES

WHAT IS A PORTION?

Knowing how much, as well as what we should eat, is vitally important in maintaining ideal body weight. It will take a little longer than following a strict diet, but you will enjoy your food and the weight loss will be long term. The foodservice industry is partly responsible for the high calories of food and the amount of food we have been eating. During the last two decades, all food portions have been super-sized. Bread used to be one-ounce per slice, but now most bakery companies make each slice 1.4 to 1.5 ounces per slice. Some bagels are large enough to make four servings of bread. In addition, potato, pasta and sandwich portions served in restaurants are two to four times larger than they were twenty years ago.

A serving of bread is one ounce, and a serving portion of pasta or rice is a ½ cup. A meat serving is not a sixteen-ounce steak; it is three to four ounces of beef, pork or chicken per serving. A serving of milk is eight-ounces, a serving of vegetable is half a cup, and a serving of fruit is the size of a peach or tangerine. Review the <u>Food Portion Charts</u> for serving sizes in this chapter. Try *measuring your food with a measuring utensil first; then empty the food on a plate, bowl or cup to visually estimate portion sizes. After a few measuring experiments you will not need the measuring utensil. Teach your children and other family members to do the same. By the way, you should own a set of measuring cups, spoons and a small scale that measures ounces.*

On a recent visit to a new Italian restaurant, which received a very good review, I was not surprised to read how large the portions were for the price charged. Most of the reviewers evaluating restaurant menus follow the same pattern; their main interest is to cover portion size, taste, price and service. No one appears to be concerned about nutrition, freshness or quality any more. Since I was writing on the subject of overeating, I decided to see for myself. My guest and I waited at the door forty-five minutes for a table, while observing the plates being served to other guests with amazement. The plates were piled high with enough food to feed a family. We decided to skip the appetizer and order a small basket of bread while we waited for the lunch entrees. The bread was served to our table consisting of half loaf with five slices of melted cheese on top. The bread alone was more than lunch for two. When the lunch entrée was served I said, "I guess we are going to be eating Italian for the next two days." Five three-inch round meatballs were placed between a 12-inch loaf of bread, topped with three slices of cheese and tomato sauce served with a huge portion of fried potatoes. Each meal contained more than the calories we needed for the entire day. Unless you are a 6'2" man who works construction, who can really eat this much food? Many of us do because we don't want to waste it and that, is a big mistake.

As a restaurant owner, I have observed people eating a lot of food in one meal. More than half of the people eating in full service restaurants can easily eat an appetizer, salad, dinner and dessert. In addition, we are attracted to advertisements promoting a lot of food for a little money. We may be saving a few dollars, but later we pay for it in weight loss programs and doctors visits. Fast food restaurants entice us with advertising phrases such as "all you can eat," "the jumbo burger," "free fries," "free soda," "all you can drink soda," "two pizzas for the price of one," everything is super-sized. The last thirty years, the food service industry has been partly responsible for the current problems of obesity. Only a small portion of the population eats the correct portions when eating out. Solving this problem, when such a powerful industry promotes large amounts of high fat and high calorie foods, is an individual's endeavor.

Be smart and more persistent about anything that may contribute to a health risk. Ask for healthier options in restaurants, fast food establishments, snack bars, movie theatres and food stands. As the number of requests for healthy options increase, foodservice proprietors will make them available in an effort to please the customer, as everything in business translates to profit! Another way is to write to your State Legislators and emphasize the need for more nutrition education, starting with first grade. Take charge of your health, your family's health and show some responsibility for your community.

KNOW YOUR PORTION SIZES

Instead of counting fat grams and calories, which is time consuming and can cause a constant preoccupation with food, use servings portions as a guide. Portion Tables 1-9 list the serving portion sizes for each food group. Choose foods from all the food groups and eat only the recommended servings. Unless a person is a body builder or heavy laborer, it is not necessary to eat additional servings.

Complex carbohydrates are very important to good health. Carbohydrates from legumes, green leafy vegetables, fruits and whole grain are rich in nutrients that are essential to life; but we only need a certain amount, anything beyond what we need turns into body fat. Make it a habit of eating bread without butter, and if you want something with it, try low-fat hard cheese; it may have fat, but it also provides additional nutrients such as calcium and protein. Avoid eating deep fried foods; instead, sauté the food in a small amount of extra virgin olive oil, it will taste better and will be much healthier. Add more fish to the diet; most fish is low in fat, very high in nutrients and low in calories. When purchasing meat products, look for the lean cuts and have the butcher trim the fat off all the visible fat. In addition, you can reduce the saturated fat from poultry products by removing the skin and fat before cooking. Experimenting with cooking herbs is an excellent way to enhance the flavor of foods without using a lot of fat. The recipes in the cookbook section are prepared with fresh foods, extra virgin olive oil and fresh herbs to produce meals that are delicious and satisfying.

If you must purchase snacks for an occasional consumption, such as crackers, potato chips, popped corn, tortillas and other snacks of this type; <u>read the label</u> and choose the products that provide less than 150 total calories per serving, are low in sodium (<150 mg), have less than 15% of the total calories from fat, and count the snack serving as part of the bread portion. When eating in restaurants, order sauces and dressings on the side, and use only a tablespoon. Another good way to reduce your calories is to eat the vegetable and salad first, leaving the high calorie items last. The low calorie items may satisfy you and you may stop eating. If the portions are too large, eat the correct portions and take the leftover food home, or <u>leave just it</u>. Remember that it is not the foodservice industry's responsibility to protect our health. We must take the responsibility as individuals.

"To indulge is okay, if you never had to be sorry."
-Andisthenis

Portion Sizes

TABLE 1

MEAT & POULTRY SERVING PORTIONS

Choose 2 servings Three Time Per Week

LOW-FAT

(One serving contains 21 g protein, 9 g fat and 165 calories per 3 ounce serving)

Cooked lean beef chuck, flank, tenderloin or round.

Cooked lamb leg, rib, sirloin, loin, shank or chops (with visible fat trimmed before cooking).

Cooked veal leg, loin, rib, shank or cutlet.

Cooked boneless chicken with the skin removed prior to cooking.

Cooked fish filet, clams, oysters, or shrimp.

MEDIUM-FAT

(One serving contains 21 g protein, 15 g fat, and 220 calories per 3 ounce serving)

Cooked ground beef with less than 15% fat.

Cooked pork loin, tenderloin, shoulder arm shoulder blade and Canadian bacon.

Cooked liver or sweetbreads; both are high in cholesterol.

High Fat

(One serving contains 21 g protein, 24 grams fat and 300 calories per 3 ounce serving)

>Cooked beef brisket, corned beef and ground beef (with 20% fat content).

>Commercially ground chuck, roasts or rib steaks.

>Cooked lamb breast, pork country ribs, back ribs and ground pork.

>Cooked veal breast, capon, domestic duck and goose.

TABLE 2

LEGUME SERVING PORTIONS

Choose 2 servings three times/week		
One serving portion of cooked legumes = ½ cup		
	Calories	**Protein (g)**
Lentils	105	8
Northern beans	105	7
Kidney beans	115	7.5
Navy beans	105	7
Split Peas	115	8
Garbanzo beans	110	6

TABLE 3

SEAFOOD SERVING PORTIONS

Choose a fish instead of red meat as often as possible.

Saltwater Fish

Serving Portion = 3 Ounces

	Protein (g)	**Calories**	**Fat (g)**
Bluefish	20	124	4.2
Flounder	18.8	91	1.2
Grouper	19	92	1
Halibut	20	110	<1
Ahi Tuna	23	108	2.3
Herring (Atlantic)	18	158	9
Mackerel (Atlantic)	18.6	205	20
Ocean Catfish	17.6	103	3.6
Ocean Perch	18	94	1.6
Orange Roughy	14.7	126	7
Salmon			
Chinook	20	180	10
Coho	21	146	6
Pink	20	116	3.5
Sockeye	21	168	8.5
Sea Bass	18	97	2
Sea Trout	16.7	104	3.5
Snapper	20	100	1.3
Sole	19	91	1.2
Striped Bass	17	97	2.3
Swordfish	20	121	4
Tuna (albacore)	25	177	7.6
Whitefish	19	134	5.8
Whiting	18	90	1.3

TABLE 3

SEAFOOD SERVING PORTIONS CONTINUED

FRESH WATER FISH

Serving Portions = 3 Ounces

	Protein (g)	**Calories**	**Fat (g)**
Catfish	18	116	4.25
Lake Trout	21	148	6.6
Northern Pike	19	88	.7
Rainbow Trout	20.5	118	3.3
Smelt	17.6	97	2.4
Tilapia	18	98	2.4
Walleye Pike	19	93	1.2

SHELLFISH & MOLLUSKS

Serving Portion = 3 Ounces

Clams (raw)	12.7	74	<1
Crab (Blue)	18	86	<1
Dungeness	17.4	86	<1
King	18.2	84	<1
Snow	18.5	90	1
Crayfish	18.6	89	1
Lobster	20	110	1.5
Scallops	16.7	88	<1
Shrimp	20	106	1.75
Squid (calamari)	15.5	92	1.38

Table 4

Dairy Serving Portions

Choose 2-3 low-fat portions dairy/day

Serving Portion	Protein	Fat	Calories
1 cup skim milk	9	0	90
1 cup milk (1%)	11	2.5	120
1 cup milk (2%)	10	5	130
1 cup whole milk	8	8	150
1 cup non-fat yogurt	12	0	120
1 cup cream line yogurt	8	10	160
1 cup low-fat cottage cheese	14	2	90
½ cup regular cottage cheese	14	5	120
1 ounce aged cheddar cheese	7	10	120
1 ounce sharp cheddar	7	9	110
1 ounce low- Swiss	9	3.5	70
1 ounce Swiss	9	8	110
1 ounce Munster cheese	7	9	110
1 ounce fresh goat's cheese	4	5	70
1 ounce Feta cheese	4	6	70
1 ounce Mozzarella	6	6	90
1 ounce low-fat Mozzarella	8	5	80
1 ounce Myzithra	4	6	80

"Happiness is not in the food, but in the measure"
   ____Euripides

TABLE 5

VEGETABLES SERVING PORTIONS

Choose 4-6 servings/day
(Each serving contains 2 g protein, 5 g carbohydrates, <50 calories per serving, and no fat)

One serving portion = ½ cup

Asparagus	Beet Greens
Beets	Green Chard
Broccoli	Collard Greens
Cabbage	Dandelion Greens
Carrots	Spinach
Cauliflower	Turnip Greens
Eggplant	Bean Sprouts
Green Pepper	Water Chestnuts
Red & Yellow Pepper	Onions
Okra	Mushrooms
Rhubarb	Sauerkraut
Summer Squash	Tomatoes
Turnips	Zucchini

TABLE 6

STARCHY VEGETABLES SERVING PORTIONS

Each serving provides approximately 2 g protein, between 70-100 calories and 18-20 g carbohydrates

One cooked serving portion is:

½ cup of lima beans	½ cup of winter squash
½ cup of fresh peas	½ cup of yams
1 small potato	¼ cup of sweet potato
¾ cup of pumpkin	

Table 7

Fruit Serving Portions

(Each serving contains approximately 10 grams of carbohydrates and 40 calories)

Choose 4 servings/day

One serving is:

1	small apple
2	medium apricots
1	small nectarine
1	small orange
1	small pear
½	grapefruit
¾	cup strawberries
½	cup blueberries or blackberries
¼	small cantaloupe
½	cherries or grapes
1	cup of cut melon
½	small mango
½	cup fresh pineapple
1	small tangerine
1/3	cup cider or apple juice
½	cup orangc or grapcfruit juicc
¼	cup prune or grape juice
½	cup cranberry juice
4	dried apricots
2	dates or 1 fig
2	tablespoons of raisins

"Unlike most people who live to eat, I eat to live"
-Socrates

TABLE 8

BREAD & CEREAL SERVING PORTIONS

(1 serving of bread or cereal should contain approximately 90-120 calories, 18-20 g of carbohydrates, 2-5 g of protein and < .5 grams fat)

One serving portion is:

1-ounce slice of white bread
1-ounce slice of wheat bread
1-ounce slice of rye bread
1 six-inch tortilla
½ English muffin
6 baked crackers
1 ounce French roll
6 small wonton wraps
½ of a small bagel
½ pita
1 cup puffed cereal
½ cup cooked cereal
½ cup cooked barley
½ cup cooked pasta
3 cups popped popcorn
½ cup bran flakes
½ cup cooked rice
2 tablespoons dry corn meal

Some prepared bread and cereal products contain more fat, sugar, and calories **(read the label!)**

Table 9

Nut Serving Portions

One serving = ¼ cup

	Calories	**Protein (g)**	**Fat (g)**
Black walnuts	195	6.5	18.5
Pecans	202	3	21
Peanuts	210	9	18
Almonds	193	6	17.5
Roasted Cashews	196	6	16

Try to avoid consuming these Saturated fats:

Butter
Bacon fat
Bacon
Cream
Sour cream
Heavy cream
Cream cheese
Coconut

French dressing
Creamed cheese dressing
Ranch dressing
Mayonnaise
Salt pork
Sesame oil
Coconut cream

Two tablespoons of added fat a day can translate to as much as 22 pounds of added body fat in one year!

"A small amount is good and precious in all things, including food."
                                                            -Eriphos

HAVE THE FOLLOWING FOODS AVAILABLE FOR A "SNACK ATTACK"

- *Frozen or fresh berries.*
- *Fresh citrus fruit or juice.*
- *Fresh melons, peaches or plums.*
- *Plain or roasted walnuts, almonds or other nuts that do not contain sugar or high amounts of salt.*
- *Peanut butter.*
- *Dried fruit.*
- *Baked crackers with less than 120 calories per serving and less than 10% fat.*
- *Toasted pita bread.*
- *Hard cheese.*
- *Low-fat milk.*
- *Low-fat cottage cheese.*
- *Low-fat plain yogurt.*
- *Hardboiled eggs.*
- *Cut fresh vegetables.*
- *Fresh tomatoes.*

Remember to always limit consumption to one portion, and give yourself some time, before you eat another portion.

CHAPTER 6

THE BENEFITS OF AN ACTIVE LIFE

Keeping the extra weight off is not easy, that is why it is so important to develop healthy habits early in life, and make a commitment to practice self-control and persistence. Living an active life is an important factor in controlling your weight and reducing the risk of many diseases. Exercise, combined with deep breathing, floods the body with oxygen promoting an antioxidant effect that fights against disease.

Don't just think about exercise, <u>do it!</u> <u>Start now, today and for the rest of your life</u>. You are never too old or too young to start. Exercise helps you lose weight and helps maintain it, improves muscle strength and tone, improves heart and lung function, normalizes your blood pressure, and reduces the risk of diabetes and heart disease. From the beginning of your exercise routine you will notice the benefits; you will feel more energized and alert, more able to deal with daily stress situations, have a more restful sleep and in addition, you will feel good about the way you look.

There are two types of exercise activities, **aerobic** *and* **anaerobic.** *To convert fat into energy one needs to do aerobic exercises or activities that require oxygen to burn fat as the fuel for the activity. In aerobic exercise, the duration or length of time of the activity is more important than the intensity. An hour walk is considered an aerobic exercise, but running a ten-meter dash is an anaerobic exercise and it uses muscle or liver glycogen stores for energy. Jogging, cycling, swimming, dancing, tennis, walking, gymnastics and volleyball are good examples of aerobic exercise. Walking is the best form of exercise; it is easy to do, it can be done at any age with a good pair of walking shoe, and easily accessible and effortable. However, before you start an exercise program, consider making realistic goals that will enable you to stick to the program.*

Answer the following questions:

- *Will you enjoy the activity you have decided to start?*
- *Will you feel safe doing it?*
- *Is the activity easily accessible?*
- *Is the activity a part of your daily schedule?*
- *Is the activity within you financial means?*
- *Do you have any physical limitations that would prevent you from doing the activity?*
- *Did you discuss your physical activity plan with your doctor?*

If the answer is "yes" to all of the above questions, your activity program will be long-term and you will succeed!

APPROXIMATE CALORIES USED AS FUEL IN ONE HOUR FOR PEOPLE BETWEEN 120-200 LBS

ACTIVITY	CALORIES USED/HOUR
Aerobic Dance	250-500
Basketball	550-900
Cycling (10mph)	550-900
Swimming (laps)	550-900
Jogging (6mph)	550-900
Tennis	550-900
Walking (4mph)	250-420
Volleyball	150-300

MUSCLE FITNESS

Muscle strength exercises increase muscle tissue and reduce excess fat by burning a large number of calories. Training with weights uses up an average of 600 calories per hour, depending on body size, and is the most commonly used method for developing muscle and strength. Dumbbells, barbells and weight training machines are used for resistance.

Muscle strength and stretching exercises can be done without the cost of a health club, by using the body's own muscle strength and resistance.

Isometric exercises can also build muscle and strength, accomplished by tightening the muscle and holding it in position, relaxing and repeating. Additionally, these exercises can be done by applying pressure with one body part against another, or against another object. Muscle strength exercises should be done every other day to give the muscle a chance to recover. Stretching however, can be done every day, especially after waking up in the morning. Stretching exercise can use up an average of 300 calories per hour. Taking a few minutes before dressing for work to stretch, will be rewarding and worth your time.

PROPER HYDRATION

Water makes up sixty percent of our weight and is required for all the chemical reactions that take place within our body. Dehydration has serious implications, and is a major contributor to disease and headaches. Therefore, proper hydration is essential to good health. Make a habit of drinking a glass of water before and after bedtime to restore water losses occurring during sleep, drink water before meals to help with digestion and promote fullness. In addition, you should have a water bottle in your car or office and drink water before drinking anything else. During exercise, <u>water is the most important nutrient</u>; drink water before, during and after exercise, especially when doing intense activities such as jogging or hiking. The longer the duration and intensity of the exercise, the more water is needed to burn calories.

Relaxation

Relaxation is just as important to health as exercise and we need a balance of both. Deep breathing is an effective relaxation technique using the abdomen to inhale and exhale deeply, sending new oxygen supply to the lungs, and thus reducing muscle tension and heart rate. If you feel sleepy during working hours, it may be from lack of oxygen due to poor circulation, to re-energize; try deep breathing for a few minutes. Deep breathing promotes alertness during the day and good restful sleep at night.

Visualization is a helpful technique used to promote relaxation. Find a quiet place and close your eyes, giving yourself permission to escape for a few minutes; imagine being in a beautiful place, surrounded by wonderful smells and sounds, blocking out any stressful thoughts. Think of a beautiful beach at sunset, the sound of the waves, the singing of birds in the garden, the smell of gardenias or a soft breeze on you face.

ACTIVITIES TO HELP YOUR BODY USE CALORIES EFFICIENTLY

Choose an aerobic activity that you enjoy and stay with it for the rest of your life.

Do muscle strength exercises thirty minutes a day three times a week; and, walk for an hour four times per week.

Use the stairs instead of an elevator.

Take walking and stretching breaks at work for 5-10 minutes.

Cleaning the house utilizes 300 calories per hour. Mopping the floor, cleaning the windows and vacuuming are a good aerobic exercise.

Walk your dog for 30 minutes daily, instead of letting the dog out.

Park your car a few blocks away from a restaurant and walk a couple of blocks before and after dinner.

Plan to take routine walks with a friend or family member. It can be a great time for bonding.

The Benefits of an Active Live

HEIGHT & WEIGHT TABLE FOR WOMEN
AGES 25-59

Height in Feet & Inches	Small Frame	Medium Frame	Large Frame
4'10"	97-106	104-116	113-126
4'11"	98-108	106-119	115-129
5'0"	99-110	108-121	117-132
5'1"	101-113	110-124	120-135
5'2"	105-116	113-127	123-138
5'3"	106-119	116-130	125-142
5'4"	109-121	119-133	129-146
5'5"	112-125	122-136	132-150
5'6"	115-128	125-139	135-154
5'7"	118-131	128-142	138-158
5'8"	121-134	131-145	141-162
5'9"	124-138	134-148	144-165
5'10"	127-140	137-151	147-168
5'11"	133-146	140-154	150-171

Approximate weights in pounds according to frame size, without clothes or shoes, weighed in the morning. Based on lowest mortality and revised from the Met Life Charts 1999.

HEIGHT & WEIGHT TABLE FOR MEN
AGES 25-59

Height in Feet & inches	Small Frame	Medium Frame	Large Frame
5'2"	125-131	128-138	135-148
5'3"	127-133	130-140	137-151
5'4"	129-135	132-143	139-155
5'5"	131-137	134-146	141-159
5'6"	133-140	137-149	144-163
5'7"	135-143	140-152	147-167
5'8"	137-146	143-155	150-171
5'9"	139-149	146-158	153-175
5'10"	141-152	149-161	154-179
5'11"	144-155	152-165	159-183
6'	147-159	155-169	163-187
6'1"	150-163	159-173	167-192
6'2"	153-167	166-177	171-197
6"3"	157-171	169-182	176-202

Approximate weights in pounds according to frame size, without clothes or shoes, weighed in the morning. Based on lowest mortality and revised from the Met Life Charts, 1999

How To Determining Your Calorie Needs

Basal Metabolic Energy (BMR) factor for men is 1 calorie for kilogram of body weight per hour.

Basal Metabolic Energy (BMR) factor for women is .9 calories for kilogram of body weight per hour.

Example: Calculate the BMR of a woman who weighs 130 pounds

Step 1 Convert pounds to kilograms

130 lb divided by 2.2 lbs per kilogram = 59 kilograms

Step 2 Multiply weight in kilograms by BMR factor

59 kilogram X .9 = 53 calories per hour

Step 3 Multiply the calories used in one hour by the hours in one day

53 calories per hour X 24 hours = 1272 BMR calories

Step 4 to determine total calories needed for physical activity multiply the BMR calories by .10 (10 percent for sedentary lifestyle) and add to BMR calories

      1272 X .10 = 127
      1272 + 127 = 1399

Step 5 add 10% on the total from step four for energy used during the ingestion of food

> 1399 X .10 = 139 calories
> 1399 + 139 = 1538
>
> 1538 is the total calories needed per day to maintain the weight of a woman who weighs 130 lbs and who is not active.

FACTORS USED FOR ACTIVITY LEVELS

Activity	**BMR +**
Sedentary life, mostly seating	+ 10%
Exercises 3 times per week (1 hour)	+ 20%
Exercises every day (1 hour)	+ 30%
Construction worker or body builder	+40%

Remember to subtract 5% from the total calories for each decade after the age of twenty.

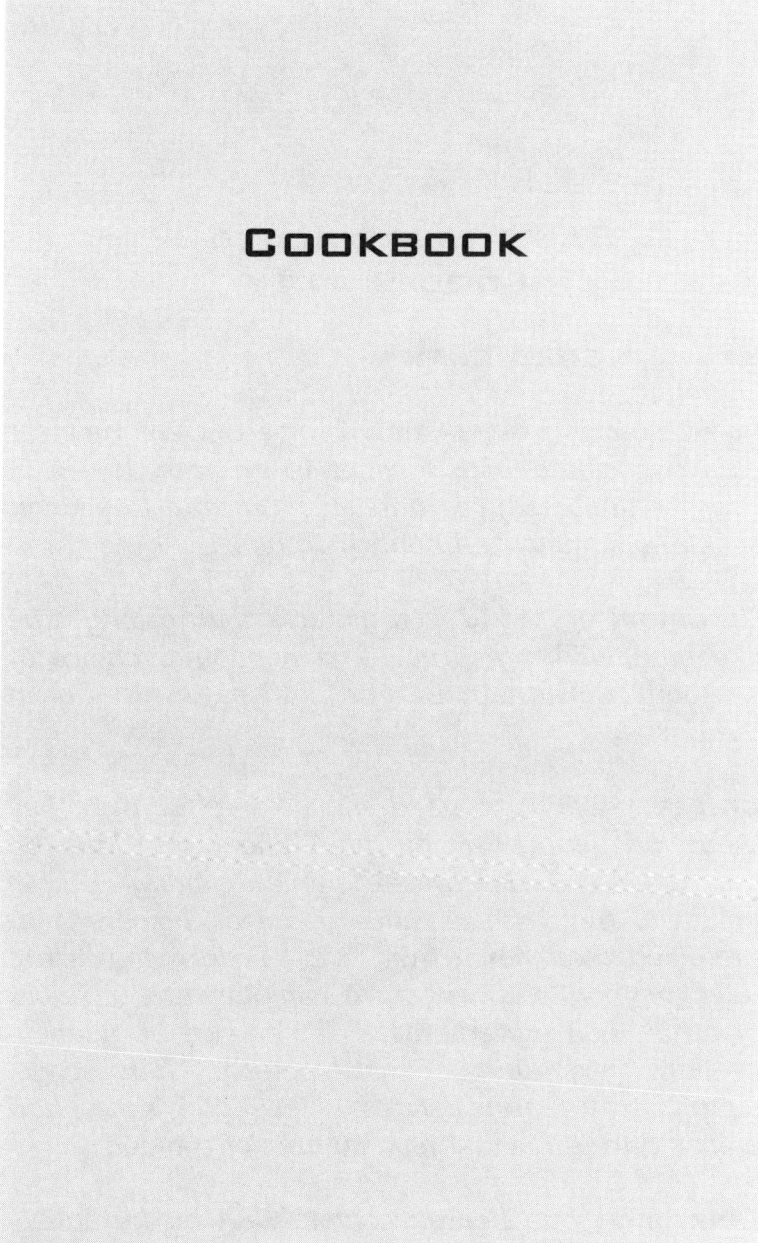

CHAPTER 7

BASIC INGREDIENTS & FOOD SAFETY

BASIC INGREDIENTS

Basil *means kingly, and during ancient times it was associated with love. It is an aromatic herb used to flavor sauces and stuffing, and to season vegetables, meat and poultry dishes.*

Calamari or squid *is a mollusk with a long tube like body with ten arms. It is a popular choice of seafood in Southern Europe, and more recently in the U.S.*

Chives *have been used in cooking for over five thousand years, first by the Chinese and later by the Greeks. In ancient times, many people believed that chives have magical powers that protected their home from evil. Today, chives are used in food preparation to compliment the flavor of other food ingredients. Chives can be used to prepare vegetables, meat, poultry, fish, eggs, soups, sauces and stews. For full flavor, add chives during the last few minutes of cooking.*

Cinnamon *has been recommended by herbalists to help with digestion problems. Japanese studies* showed that a compound in cinnamon destroys bacteria and fungi, including the bacteria causing botulism poisoning, staph infection and poisonous carcinogens. Cinnamon is an important ingredient to many culturally diverse cuisines around the world, used to prepare meats and dessert dishes. Cinnamon is available in whole sticks or ground.

Cloves are used in cooking, to freshen the breath and to relieve toothache (by holding a bruised clove in the mouth around the area of the pain). In food preparation, cloves are used to flavor meats stews, fruit pies, sweet bread, spiced tea, pudding and pickling brines.

Coriander is an herb used for over 3000 years and believed to have aphrodisiac powers that arouse passion. Coriander has been used to cure an upset stomach and as an aid to digestion. It has a bold sage flavor and a taste of citrus favored by Southeast Asia, Chinese, East India, South America, Spain and Mexican cuisines. The flavor of coriander combines well with sausage, clams, oysters and potato dishes. It can also be used to flavor marinades and salad dressing.

Dill is an ancient herb with a dominant flavor often used by European and American herbalists for relief from flatulence, to increase mother's milk and to relieve baby's colic. The dill seeds are used to flavor breads, while the leaves are used in salads, vegetables, fish, meat, poultry, soups, sauces and dressings.

Fennel is an anise-flavored herb that looks like a celery stalk used by British herbalists for weight reduction. The seeds were used as an appetite suppressant during medieval fasting periods. In food preparation fennel can be used to flavor desserts, breads, fish, sausage, duck, cabbage, beets, potatoes, lentils and cheese. Fennel is available as fresh, dried or ground.

Feta (originally from Greece) is a white semi-soft salty cheese made from goats, sheep's or cow's milk. Excellent on salads, baked vegetable dishes and pies.

Garlic is a health culinary herb with an extraordinary taste and smell, loved by most people and widely used to flavor all foods, except desserts. During ancient times it was eaten as a vegetable and not as a condiment. In the U.S., garlic lovers have even formed a club, and some people believe that garlic has magical powers against evil. In ancient Egypt it was believed that eating garlic increases strength and endurance. Throughout the world garlic has been used to cure parasites, high blood pressure and help prevent some types of cancer.

Ginger has been used for over four hundred years. The Greeks were the first to use ginger in bread baking and the Spanish conquistadors introduced it to the New World. By late 1800s ginger was a popular culinary herb in Europe. More recently, it has been used to aid digestion and to relieve problems with flatulence. As a culinary herb, ginger is used to flavor many dishes in China, Japan, Southeast Asia, North Africa, India and the Caribbean. In the U.S., it is used to flavor sweet potatoes, stuffing, poultry, quick breads, pumpkin, rhubarb, sweet pudding, cakes, cookies and muffins. It is available fresh, as dried pieces and ground. To maintain flavor, wrap tightly and store in the refrigerator.

Grape leaves are packed in jars with brine and they should be rinsed under cold running water before using. Grape leaves can be stuffed with meat or a mixture of rice and herbs.

Kaseri is a semi-soft cheese from Greece made from goat's milk. It is used on salads, for sautéing or just to eat plain.

Kalamata Olives are dark purple to black in color and are primarily produced in the southern mainland of Greece. Kalamata olives can be found in most supermarkets packaged in jars or cans.

Lemons and their juice are frequently used in Greek cooking. Fresh squeezed lemons are used to flavor or marinate steaks, pork chops, grilled chicken, lamb chops, soups and sauces.

Marjoram was allegedly called the "precious herb" by Aphrodite, the goddess of love, and was used by the ancient Greeks to cure rheumatism. It was also used as medicine to cure minor health problems with asthma, indigestion, toothache and eye infections. Marjoram is used in cooking to flavor meats, poultry, fish, pates, vegetables, stews, sauces, butter, and to flavor vinegar and oil.

Mint was considered by the Greeks a symbol of hospitality and was also used to cure soar throat, insomnia, headache, heartburn, hiccups, colic, indigestion, flatulence, to freshen breath and temporarily reduce hunger. Mint ranges from mild spearmint to strong peppermint. The peppermint is used to flavor candy, beverages and gum. The spearmint variety is used to flavor meats, fish, poultry, vegetables and legumes. Mint is available fresh, dried leaves and extracts.

Myzithra is a salty and hard white cheese made from goat's milk, used mostly as grated cheese.

Nutmeg is the dried seed found inside the tropical fruit of a nutmeg tree used to flavor meat and poultry dishes, sauces, muffins, breads and cookies. It is available whole or ground.

Onion. The white onion has strong pungent flavor, while the yellow is milder and sweeter. Onion is the plant that Alexander The Great fed his troops to give them strength and endurance for battle. Greeks and Italians use onion in most of their dishes. Onion is the most commonly used and best liked vegetable/herb in the world! And except for desserts, onions have unlimited possibilities in food preparation.

Oregano is a very potent antioxidant, and the most fragrant grows in the mountains of Greece, hence the translation for its name, which means "joy of the mountains" in Greek. It was the Greeks and Romans who first used oregano as medicine, as well as in cooking. Unaware of oregano's antioxidant properties at the time, the ancient Greeks used oregano as tea to cure chronic cough, asthma and to relieve muscle aches. Oregano did not catch on in cooking until the nineteenth century and after World War II, when our servicemen returned from Italy with an acquired taste for pizza and oregano. Since then, oregano was adopted as America's favorite herb; the aromatic herb with a hot and peppery flavor is very popular in food preparation and is used to season salads, meats, fish, poultry, omelets, quiches, sauces and breads.

Parsley comes in two varieties, curly and flat; both varieties have a gentle flavor and fragrance. Parsley is among the most commonly used herbs for cooking and garnishing. The Greeks used parsley to decorate wreaths worn by athletes after winning, and also fed it to racehorses in order to promote stamina and endurance. During the middle ages parsley was used to fight against asthma, jaundice, plaque and to relieve digestion and constipation symptoms. Today, it is used for its delicate flavor and nutritional properties.

Phyllo is a pastry made from wheat flour into very thin pastry layers. Each pastry leaf is 12X20 inches and is packed in one-pound packages. The best way to defrost phyllo pastry is in the refrigerator overnight.

Rosemary grows as a bush in almost any garden. During the ancient times, it was used to treat depression, headaches, muscle spasms, and to fight against bacterial infections. However, large quantities of the concentrated oil may harm the stomach, intestines and kidneys. The flavor of this herb compliments poultry, fish, meats and wild game dishes. It is also used to make breads, cream sauces, soups, marinades and dressings. Rosemary is available fresh, whole dried and ground.

Semolina is a high protein wheat product used to make puddings, bread and pasta products.

Souvlaki is small pieces of meat marinated in olive oil, lemon juice and herbs, and then grilled.

Tarragon has a very delicate flavor and an important ingredient in stocks and sauces; it is considered to be one of the finest herbs, which was originally used in France. Tarragon is widely used to flavor and enhance the taste of salads, sauces, dressings, meats, poultry, fish and vegetables. When added to cooked products, add tarragon the last few minutes of cooking for full flavor without bitterness. Tarragon is available fresh or dried and best when stored in the freezer.

Thyme has a delicate taste of clove and it is considered one of the finest herbs in the French cuisine used to flavor soups, sauces, gravies and stuffing. This herb grows in abundance in the island of Hydra, Greece and in the past it has been used as an antiseptic and a pain reliever. Thyme is available fresh, dried and in oil. In its pure form, thyme oil can be toxic and may cause dizziness, *diarrhea, nausea and vomiting, headache and muscular weakness.*

Tomatoes *are almost always a part of the dinner table in Greece and because of their great taste and nutritional content they are an important ingredients in the preparation of many dishes around the world. Tomatoes can be used to flavor meats, poultry, seafood, soups and sauces. When fresh tomatoes are not available, tomato paste and other canned tomato products are an excellent substitute.*

Watercress *is a peppery herb rich in lenoleic acid, which is found to be beneficial in fighting heart disease. It has glossy dark green leaves and grows wildly in shallow streams. Watercress is most commonly used in salads or as a garnish.*

FOOD BORN ILLINESS

Millions of Americans suffer from food poisoning every year with symptoms similar to those associated with the common flu. In fact, people often mistake food poisoning for the "24-hour flu." Contaminated food products, pesticide residues on fruits and vegetables, and eggs contaminated with salmonella are a health threat to the public. The principal causes of food contamination are infected handlers, contaminated food supplies, unsafe handling, unsanitary equipment and hazardous chemicals. Although there is little we can do about the safety of food supplies before we bring them home, there is a lot that can be done to prevent further contamination, through proper handling and storage, after we bring perishable foods home.

Bacteria are so small that they cannot be seen by the naked eye. Approximately ten million of the tiny organisms can fit on the head of a pin. During the growth phase, bacteria can multiply to more than four thousand in one hour. Factors encouraging bacterial growth include protein, moisture, temperature and time. The presence of acid, salt and sugar inhibit bacterial growth and act as preservatives. Bacteria grow quickly in foods containing protein such as fish, poultry, eggs, milk, meat-based soups, sauces and gravies. These foods should be handled at proper temperatures to prevent bacterial growth. The danger zone for bacterial growth is between 45-140 (F) degrees, a temperature range where harmful bacteria multiply very quickly. Cold foods should be stored at temperatures below 45 F *degrees and hot foods should be kept above 140 F degrees to prevent bacteria from growing. Bacteria in foods contaminated before freezing will resume its growth during defrosting, if it is defrosted in room temperature. To prevent this, always defrost perishable foods in the refrigerator and any additional bacteria remaining can be destroyed when the food is cooked above 145 (F) degrees. The relationship between time and temperature is important in preventing bacterial growth. Food that stands at room temperature has a safety zone of two hours. After that, <u>it should be thrown away.</u>*

HANDLING SEAFOOD

Before storing fresh fish it should be gutted and rinsed under cold water and place in a strainer for a few minutes to drain excess water. For freezer storage, divide the fish in portions and place in airtight bags, pressing the air out and sealing the bags tightly. Proper wrapping will prevent dehydration and oxidation, which causes the fish to become dry, tough, and changes its texture. Mark the date on the package and store in the coldest part of the freezer.

Crustaceans include crab, lobster and shrimp. Mollusks include octopus, clams, oysters and scallops. Fresh shellfish should be alive when purchased and before cooking, but do not leave them submerged in water, as they will die. Once cooked, their color turns bright red and has a mild odor. Seafood products are highly perishable and should be cooked or stored immediately. If seafood is purchased fresh, it can be stored in the refrigerator between 32-40 F. up to three days. Since seafood has little or no connective tissue, it requires very little cooking to become tender. On the other hand, if fish is overcooked, it will become tough and dry.

REFRIGERATOR & FREEZER STORAGE FOR SEAFOOD

RAW SEAFOOD	REFRIGERATOR	FREEZER
Fresh Fish (lean)	2-5 days	2-6 months
Fresh Fish (Medium fat)	2-3 days	2-3 months
Live Lobster	1-3 days	2-3 months
Live Mussels	4-5 days	3-4 months
Live Oysters	7-10 days	3-4 months
Live Crab	3-5 days	2-3 months
Canned Crab (Pasteurized)	6 months	
Canned Crab (After opening)	3-5 days	
Scallops	2-3 days	3-4 months
Squid (whole)	2-3 days	1-2 months
Squid (cleaned)	3-4 days	3-4 months
Cooked seafood	3-4 days	
Smoked seafood	4-5 days	

Cookbook: Basic Ingredients and Food Safety

HANDLING POULTRY AND EGGS

When purchasing poultry, make sure that it is free of bruises, blood or feathers, and the skin is plump. It should be washed thoroughly under cold running water prior to cooking and storing. Poultry products should be used in cooking within two days from purchase or placed in airtight bags for freezer storage. Poultry products are often contaminated with salmonella bacteria, therefore, it becomes very important to practice sanitary handling and storing at home. All the kitchen equipment used during food preparation should be thoroughly cleaned and sanitized immediately after handling the poultry. If a sanitizer is not available, use a bowl of water mixed with a tablespoon of bleach to sanitize. This should be done after thoroughly washing all the utensils and equipment used to prepare the food.

Eggs are also an excellent medium for bacterial growth, and while the interior portion of the eggs is sanitary, the shell is often contaminated with bacteria. When the shell brakes, it can pick up bacteria from the shell, the air, people and utensils. However, eggs should not be washed before storing in their raw form, because the added moisture enables the bacteria to penetrate the shell faster.

Tips For Safe Food Handling

Wash your hands with soap and water before preparing food.

Clean and sanitize cutting boards, can openers, knives and other utensils.

Use paper towels rather than cloth or sponge to wipe up spills.

Always thaw frozen foods in the refrigerator, especially foods containing eggs, milk, seafood, meat and poultry.

Always keep raw foods separate from cooked foods and do not leave perishable foods in room temperature for more than two hours.

Keep perishable foods in refrigerator temperatures under 40 F.

All meat and poultry products should be cooked to the minimum internal temperature of 145 F.

Monitor the cooking temperature by inserting the meat thermometer in the center of the meat, away from the bone.

When in doubt, throw it out.

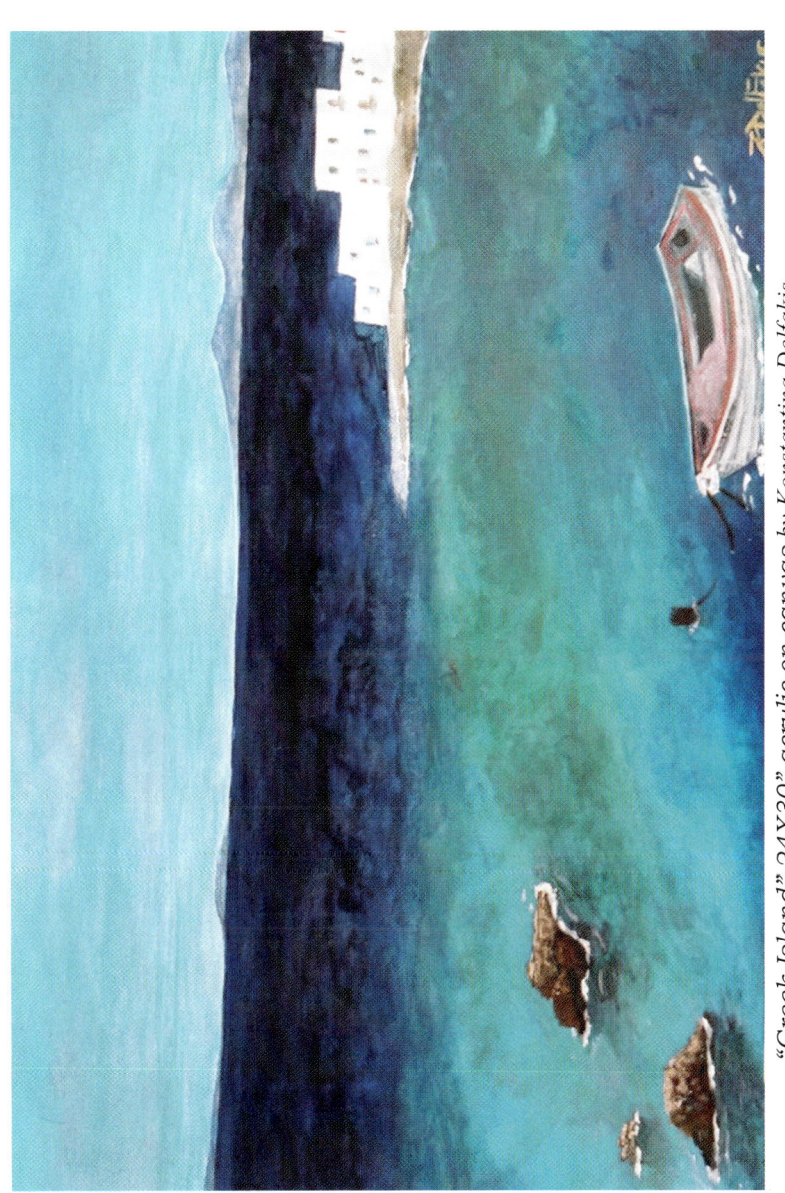

"Greek Island" 24X30" acrylic on canvas by Konstantina Delfakis

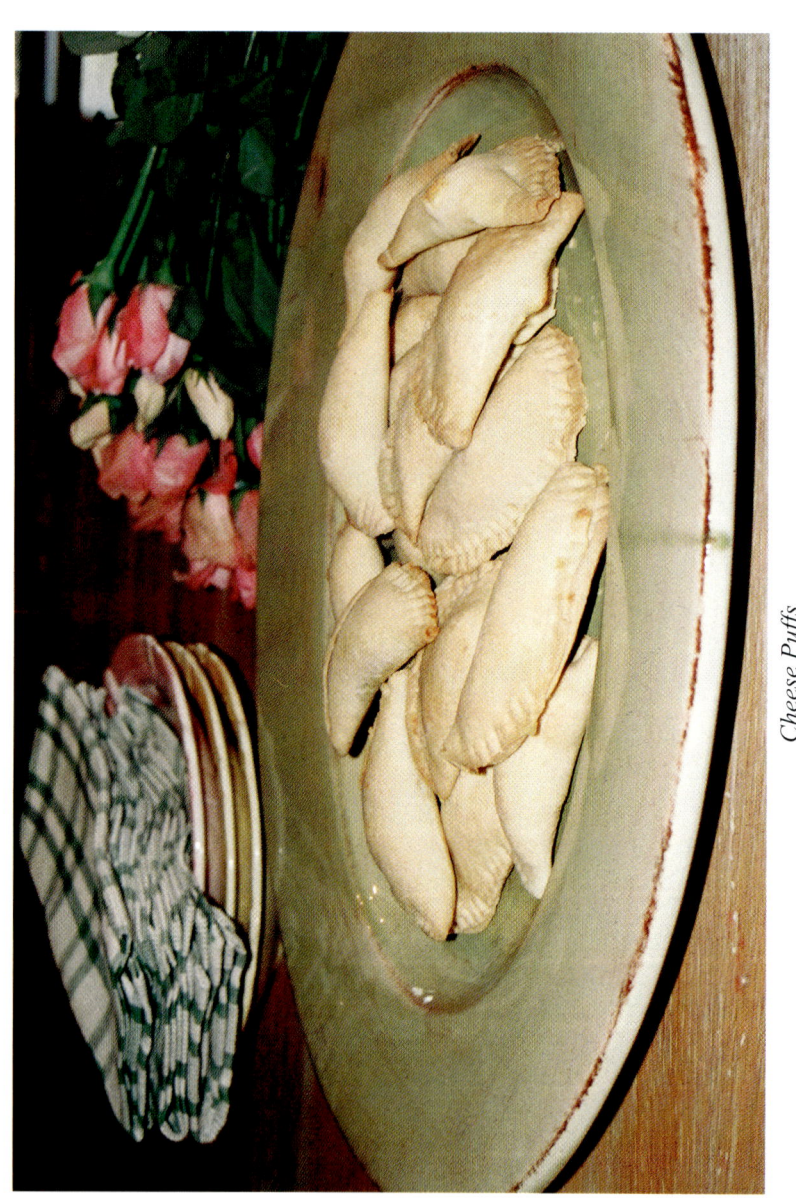
Cheese Puffs

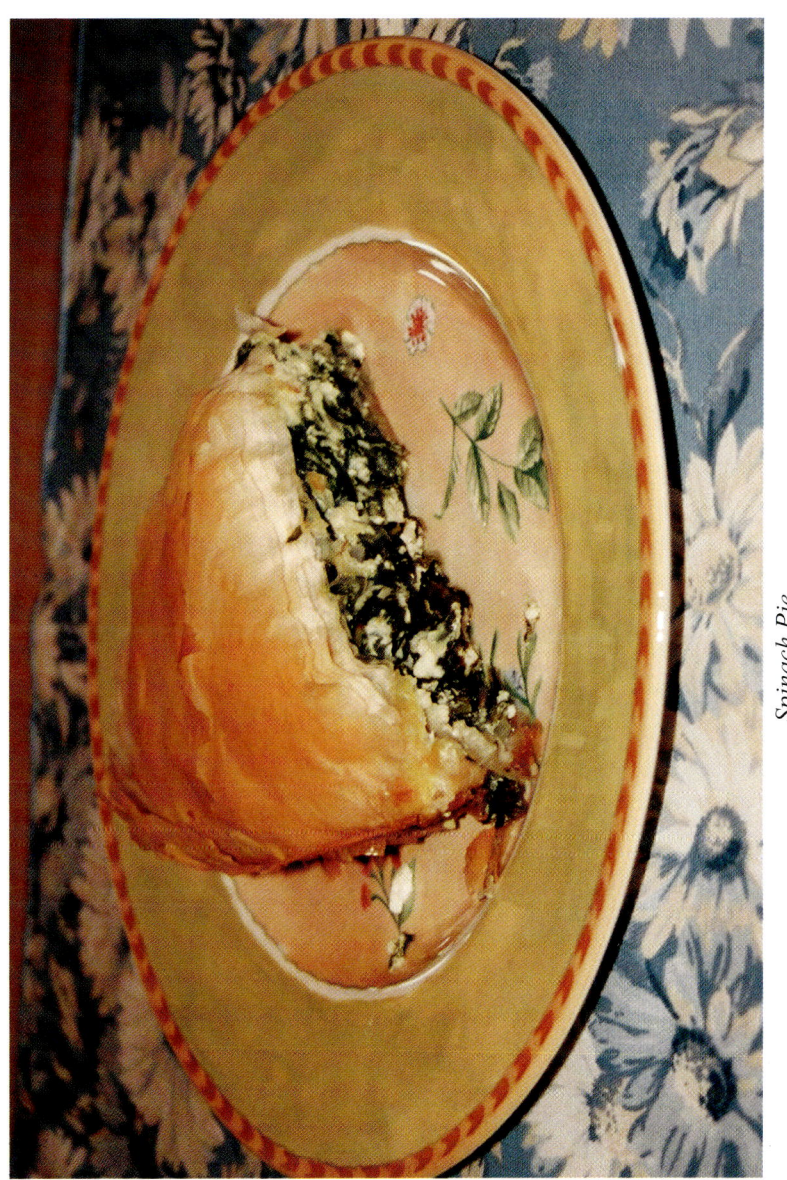

Spinach Pie

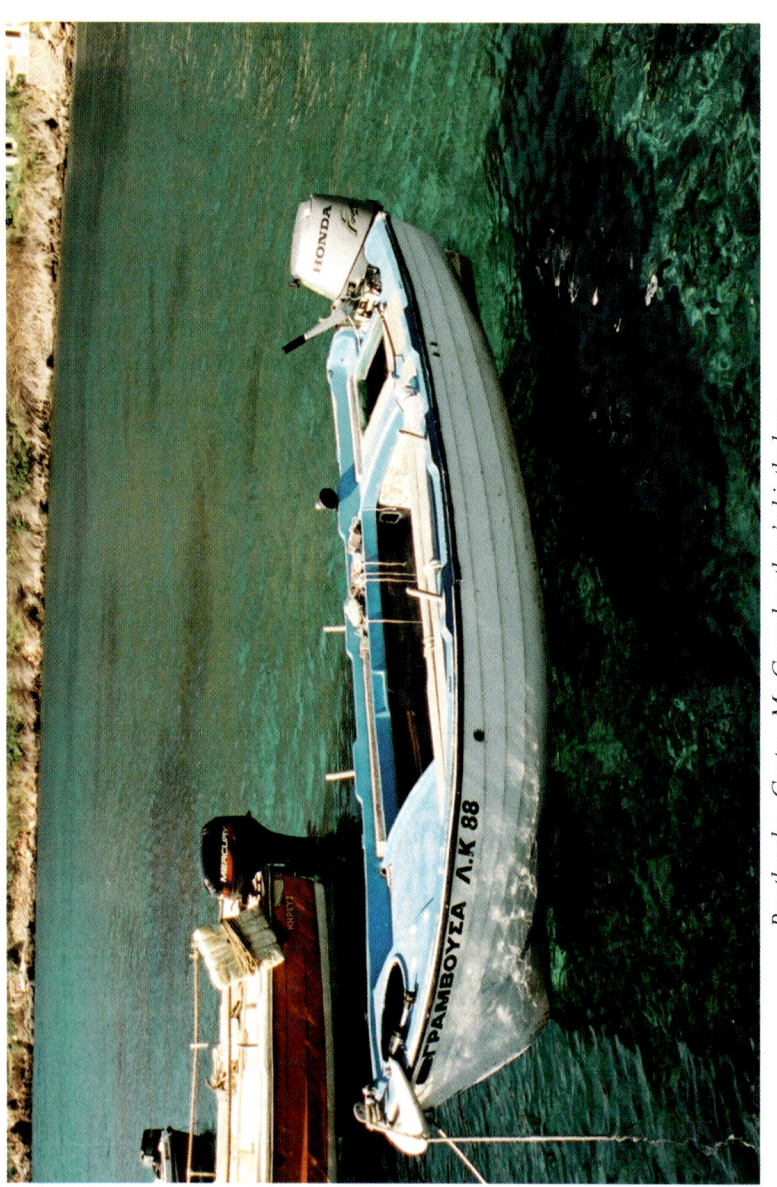

Ravthouha, Crete. My Grandmother's birthplace

CHAPTER 8

Starters

Shopping at the market in Crete

A trip to the market is a daily routine in Crete, it starts very early in the morning, and it is a way to shop for the fresh food items of the day and to socialize with friends. The market is wonderful! It is full of life with vendors shouting the specials of the day. There are fresh fruits and vegetables of the season in abundance, whole carcasses of fresh meat and poultry hanging in rows, and mountains of freshly caught fish and shellfish.

While at the market, there is no doubt that you will meet someone you known. One usually stops for a greeting and make plans to meet at town's square for coffee. The town's square is called a "platia", which is surrounded by shops and cafes, where friends and neighbors meet to exchange and discuss the news of the day.

Hardy White Bread

¼ cup lukewarm water [110-120F]
1 tablespoon active dried yeast
2 tablespoons olive oil
1 teaspoon salt
2 cups non-fat milk
5 cups all-purpose flour

Preheat the oven to 400 degrees Fahrenheit.
In a small saucepan heat the milk to scalding and cool to lukewarm. In a small bowl combine the lukewarm water, yeast, olive oil and salt, and stir to dissolve the yeast.

In a large bowl combine the lukewarm milk, two cups of the flour and yeast mixture, and beat with an electric mixture for 2 minutes. Add remaining flour, one cup at a time, mixing with your hands to form soft dough. Place dough in a large bowl; cover with a towel, and place in a warm area to rise for one hour.

Transfer the dough onto a floured surface and knead with hands for five minutes, and shape into loaves. Brush the bottom and sides of two 4X9X3 inch loaf pans with olive oil and place the loaves in the pan, cover with a towel and place in a warm place until double in size (2 hours). Bake in a preheated oven for 30 minutes. Let the bread cool before slicing. Makes 2 loaves.

Pita Bread

1½	cup lukewarm water
1	tablespoon active dry yeast
2	tablespoons extra virgin olive oil
1	teaspoon salt
3½	cups all-purpose flour

Preheat oven to 400 degrees Fahrenheit.
In a medium bowl combine the lukewarm water with the olive oil, salt, yeast, and stir to dissolve.

Add half of the flour to the yeast mixture and beat with a mixer for 1 minute. Add the remaining flour and knead into soft dough.

Let the dough rise in a warm place for 30 minutes and transfer to a floured surface.

Divide the dough in eight portions, and roll each piece into 9- inches in diameter. Place the formed pita on a lightly greased baking sheet, cover, and let it rise again for 20 minutes. Bake in the preheated oven for 15 minutes. Serves 8

Zucchini Omelet

1	cup thinly sliced zucchini
2	tablespoons chopped green onions
2	tablespoons extra virgin olive oil
2	ounces cheddar cheese, grated
4	jumbo eggs
	a pinch of salt and pepper
2	tablespoons of milk

Gather all the ingredients.

In a medium size bowl combine the eggs, milk, salt and pepper. Beat for one minute with an electric mixer or a whisk and set aside.

In a large skillet, heat the olive oil over low heat and sauté the zucchini slices with the onions until they are lightly wilted.

Add the egg mixture, quickly scraping the egg from the side of the pan to the center, as it cooks; add the grated cheese on top of the eggs, cover, and remove the pan from the heat.

Wait a few minutes before serving to allow the cheese to melt on top of the eggs. Serves 4. Serve with fresh fruit and one piece of whole-wheat toast per person.

Greek Salad

1	large head romaine lettuce
2	medium tomatoes cut into small wedges
1	European cucumber, peeled and sliced
1	small red onion, sliced thin
1	green pepper, sliced thin
	salt and pepper to taste
½	teaspoon dried Greek oregano
4	tablespoons olive oil
2	tablespoons white balsamic vinegar

Toppings:

4	ounces Feta cheese, crumbled
4	Greek peperoncini
8	Kalamata olives

Fill the kitchen sink with cold water and wash the lettuce leaf by leaf, discarding the bruised or wilted leaves. Place the lettuce leaves on a paper towel to dry and break into small pieces with your fingers. Chill one hour prior to making the salad.

In a large salad bowl combine the lettuce with the tomatoes, cucumber, onion, green pepper, salt and pepper, oregano, olive oil and vinegar. Toss to blend with the salad dressing and add the feta, peppers and olives on top. Serves 4-6

Sweet Pepper & Peach Salad

3	red sweet peppers cut in 1-inch wide slices
3	large peaches
½	teaspoon sugar
¼	cup slivered almonds
2	tablespoons extra virgin olive oil
	dash of cayenne pepper

Peel the skin off the peaches and cut into slices.

In a large skillet, heat the olive oil and sauté the red peppers for 2 minutes while stirring. Add the slivered almonds and continue stirring over medium heat for another minute.

Add the sliced peaches, season with cayenne pepper and sugar, and stir gently just until the peaches are warmed slightly. Serves 6

Village Salad

4	medium tomatoes
1	European cucumber
1	small red onion
1	small green pepper, sliced in thin strips
¼	teaspoon Greek oregano
½	teaspoon salt
8	Kalamata olives
¼	cup olive oil
4	ounces feta cheese cut in cubes
1	small avocado
	a few sprigs watercress

Peel and slice the onions, cucumbers and avocado.

Rinse tomatoes and watercress; slice the tomatoes in small pieces and break the watercress coarsely by hand.

In a large serving platter combine the tomatoes, cucumbers, watercress, peppers and onions, and season with salt, oregano and olive oil.

Toss to coat the ingredients with the dressing, and garnish with the olives, feta cheese and avocado slices. Serves 4

Winter Salad

1	medium size head of romaine lettuce
1	medium size head red or green leaf lettuce
½	cup thinly sliced red onion
¼	cup finely chopped fresh dill
1	medium size red pepper, sliced
1	cup fresh mushrooms, washed and sliced
3	tablespoons extra virgin olive oil
1	tablespoon wine vinegar
	salt and pepper to taste
3	hard-boiled eggs, chilled and sliced
2	ounces Feta cheese, crumbled

Wash the lettuce leaves thoroughly and cool in the refrigerator prior to preparing the salad.

Prepare the remaining ingredients and tear the lettuce leaves into small bite size pieces. Add the dill, pepper and mushrooms.

Season with salt, pepper, olive oil, vinegar, and toss gently to coat the ingredients with the seasonings.

Garnish the top with sliced hardboiled eggs and crumbled Feta cheese. Serves 6

Eggplant Salad

This is a wonderful summer salad served with pita

1	lb eggplant
2	cloves fresh garlic, finely chopped
2	tablespoons olive oil
2	tablespoon wine vinegar
¼	cup finely chopped fresh parsley
½	cup finely chopped red pepper
1	large ripe tomato, finely chopped
	salt and pepper to taste

Preheat oven to 350 degrees Fahrenheit.
Cut eggplant into slices and salt heavily, place into a bowl with enough water to cover the eggplant and soak for 15 minutes. Drain and cut into small pieces.

Place the chopped eggplant in small pan and bake in the preheated oven for 30 minutes or until the eggplant is soft.

Transfer the cooked eggplant from the pan into a strainer to drain excess water.

In a small serving bowl combine the eggplant with the pepper, parsley, tomato, garlic, salt and pepper, olive oil, vinegar, and mix to blend the ingredients well. Marinate for a few hours before serving. Serve on wheat toast or pita bread. Serves 4

Potato Salad

3	lbs white potatoes
½	cup chopped green onion
¼	cup chopped fresh parsley
¼	cup olive oil
1	tablespoon white balsamic vinegar
1	teaspoon prepared mustard
1	teaspoon salt
½	teaspoon pepper
1	tablespoon capers

Peel the potatoes and cut into small wedges.

Place the potatoes in a medium size pan, cover with water and cook over medium heat for 15 minutes, or until the potatoes are easily pierced with a fork. Drain, and transfer into a large bowl.

Meanwhile, prepare the dressing in a small bowl by mixing the olive oil, vinegar and mustard.

Pour dressing over the potatoes and mix to coat well with the dressing; add the salt, pepper, parsley, onions, capers, and toss gently. Serves 6

Chicken Salad

1	lb boneless chicken breast or a small whole chicken
2	tablespoons freshly squeezed lemon juice
3	tablespoons extra virgin olive oil
2	apples peeled, cored and cut in small cubes
¼	cup finely chopped green onions
2	tablespoons finely chopped fresh parsley
¼	cup finely chopped walnuts
	salt and pepper to taste

Lightly salt the breast of chicken and place in a small saucepan with a cup of water. Simmer for 20 minutes on low heat.

Chop the cooked chicken into small bite size pieces and place in a small bowl. Add the lemon juice and olive oil, and chill in the refrigerator for an hour.

In a medium bowl combine the chicken, chopped apples, onions, parsley, walnuts, salt, pepper and mix until all the ingredients are well blended.

Chill a few minutes before serving. Serve on wheat toast with sliced tomatoes. Serves 6

Lentil Soup

¼	cup olive oil
½	cup chopped yellow onion
½	cup chopped green onion
6	ounces canned tomato paste
2	quarts water
1	cup dried lentils
¼	cup chopped parsley
2	cloves garlic, peeled and sliced
½	cup finely chopped carrots
1	teaspoon salt
¼	teaspoon pepper
2	bay leaves
1	tablespoon red balsamic vinegar

In a large saucepot, heat the olive oil over medium heat and sauté the onions.

Dilute the tomato paste in the water and add it to the pot.

Bring to a boil and reduce heat to low; add the lentils, parsley, garlic, carrots, salt, pepper, bay leaves and vinegar. Simmer for two hours, stirring occasionally. Serve hot or chilled. Serves 6

Chicken Egg-Lemon Soup

For the stock:

1	4-lb chicken, cut up
4	quarts water
1	tablespoon salt
1	carrot
1	green onion
1	clove garlic
	few peppercorns

For the soup:

2	quarts stock (from above)
1	cup uncooked converted rice
½	teaspoon salt
¼	teaspoon white pepper
2	eggs, separated
1	tablespoon cornstarch diluted in
½	cup fresh squeezed lemon juice

Fill a large pot with 4 quarts of water and add the chicken. Bring the water to a boil over medium heat. Using a slotted spoon, skim off accumulated brown fat from the broth as it boils.

Add the green onion, garlic, peppercorns, salt and carrot. Lower the heat and simmer for 1 hour. Remove the stockpot from heat and using a fine sieve, strain the stock into another large pot.

Meanwhile place the cooked chicken in a bowl to cool.

Add the rice, salt and pepper to the stock pot and continue to simmer for an additional 30 minutes until the rice is tender. Remove the pot from heat.

In a mixing bowl, beat egg whites until stiff. Add yolks and continue beating with an electric mixer; while slowly adding the cornstarch, previously diluted in lemon juice.

Slowly pour the egg-lemon mixture to the broth stirring quickly for one minute to prevent the egg from curdling.

Remove the bones from the cooked chicken and cut the breast portions into bite size pieces. Add the chicken pieces to the soup and stir. Serves 6-8.

The remaining dark chicken meat can be used for chicken salad.

Bean Soup

3	quarts water
1	lb dried navy beans
1	cup chopped yellow onion
¼	cup chopped green onion
½	cup extra virgin olive oil
1	cup coarsely chopped celery
1	cup sliced carrots
3	cloves garlic, sliced
¼	cup finely chopped Italian parsley
2	mild chili peppers, finely chopped
1	teaspoon salt

Place the beans in a large bowl with 4 cups of water and soak overnight.

Heat the olive oil in a large pot over medium heat and sauté the yellow onions until golden. Add the water, salt, beans, and cook the beans over medium heat for 2 hours.

Add the green onions, celery, carrots, garlic, parsley and chili peppers.

Continue simmering over low heat for another hour or until the beans become tender. Serves 10

Potato Clam Soup

¼	cup extra virgin olive oil
½	cup finely chopped green onions
½	cup finely chopped celery leaves
2	quarts chicken stock
1	teaspoon salt
¼	teaspoons white pepper
1	cup chopped sea clams (canned)
2	lbs new red potatoes, peeled and cut in cubes
2	large cloves of garlic freshly crushed
½	cup low-fat milk
1	tablespoon cornstarch
2	tablespoons finely chopped flat parsley
1	lemon

In a large stockpot, heat the olive oil and sauté the onions with the celery for 2-3 minutes over medium heat. Add the chicken stock, salt, pepper, potatoes and crushed garlic. Cook for 20 minutes; add the clams, and simmer for 5 minutes longer.

While the soup is still over heat source, dilute the cornstarch in the milk and add it to the soup, stirring until the soup thickens. Garnish each serving with chopped parsley and a lemon wedge. Serves 8

Cheese Puffs

For the filling:

2	cup crumbled feta cheese
4	ounces fresh goats cheese
2	tablespoons finely chopped fresh mint
3	tablespoons finely chopped chives
1	tablespoon olive oil
1	egg white, slightly beaten
	dash of white pepper

For the pastry:

4	cups flour
½	teaspoon salt
2	eggs
6	tablespoons olive oil
1	cup milk

Preheat oven to 375 degrees Fahrenheit.
To make the pastry, sift the flour with the salt and set aside. In a medium mixing bowl, beat the eggs lightly using a whisk. Add the milk, olive oil and flour mixture, and knead with your hands to form soft dough.

Divide the dough in half and keep the half you are not working on covered with a towel to prevent drying. Place the dough on a lightly floured surface and roll into a thin pastry, approximately 20" in diameter.

Using a 4-inch round cookie cutter or wide rim glass, press down against the surface to cut the pastry into eighteen 4-inch round pieces of pastry. Place each piece between two pieces of wax paper and repeat the process with the remaining dough.

Heat the olive oil in a small pan and sauté the chives until slightly wilted.

In a small bowl, combine the cheeses, chives, mint, pepper and beaten egg white blending into a thick mixture.

Place a teaspoon of the cheese mixture on the one side of each pastry piece and fold the other side of the pastry over the top to cover the cheese mixture, while lining the edges to form a half moon. Press down gently with fingers to slightly flatten.

Using pastry cutter, trim the round edges of each puff to secure closure and place on a lightly greased cookie sheet. Bake in the preheated oven for 20 minutes or pan-fry in ¼ cup olive oil. Makes 36 cheese puffs. Serves 12

Egg Whites Stuffed with Liver Pate

6	eggs, hardboiled and chilled
4	ounces chicken liver, finely chopped
2	tablespoons extra virgin olive oil
4	tablespoons finely chopped yellow onion
2	tablespoon finely chopped parsley
2	tablespoons white wine
1	teaspoon fresh squeezed lemon juice
	dash of cayenne pepper
	dash of ginger
2	tablespoons freshly chopped chives
	salt and pepper to taste

Slice the hardboiled eggs in half and remove the yolks carefully not to break the egg white. Set the egg white on a platter and refrigerate.

Cut the liver in small pieces, season with salt and pepper, and sauté with the onion in the olive oil for 2 minutes. Add the wine and cook an additional minute.

Place the liver in a small bowl and using a fork, mash into a smooth mixture; add the egg yolks, fresh parsley, chives, lemon juice, cayenne pepper, ginger, and blend well.

Using a small spoon, fill the egg whites with the liver mixture and chill for two hours before serving. Serve on a toasted baguette slice. Serves 6

Sautéed Calamari

1   *lb very small whole calamari (squid)*
½   *teaspoon salt*
    dash of pepper to taste

For *sautéing*:

½   *cup flour*
¼   *cup olive oil*
2   *cloves garlic, finely chopped*

Clean the calamari by cutting the tentacles above the eyes and removing the round beak at the base of the tentacles, pushing it out with your fingers. Pull the entrails and transparent cartilage from inside the tubular body and discard. Rinse the calamari with cold water and place in a strainer with the tentacles.

Let the calamari drain in the strainer and dry well using paper towels to remove all the moisture, and season with salt, pepper, and coat well with the flour.

In a large skillet, heat the olive oil over medium heat for 1-2 minutes. Using tong, place the floured calamari in the hot oil carefully; wait until the one side is crispy and turn, add the garlic and sauté the other side to golden. Serves 4.

Stand as far as you can, during frying, moisture inside the calamari may cause hot oil to splatter.

Sautéed Meatballs

1	lb extra lean ground beef or lamb
½	cup finely chopped onion
2	cloves garlic, finely chopped
¼	cup finely chopped fresh mint
½	teaspoon dried Greek oregano
½	cup bread crumbs
½	teaspoon salt
¼	teaspoon pepper
2	egg whites
4	ounces crumbled feta cheese

For sautéing:

¼	cup olive oil
¼	cup flour

In a large bowl combine the ground meat with the onion, garlic, mint, oregano, bread crumbs, salt, pepper, egg whites and feta cheese. Mix all the ingredients by hand until they are well blended.

Shape and divide the meat mixture in 2-ounce size meatballs. Pour the flour on a plate and coat the meatballs lightly with flour, dusting off the excess flour.

In a large skillet, heat the oil over medium heat and fill the skillet with the meatballs. Saute both sides until golden brown. Serves 6

Zucchini Croquettes

2	lbs zucchini, stems cut off and cleaned
1	large potato
¼	cup finely chopped Italian parsley
4	ounces crumbled Feta cheese
¼	cup plain breadcrumbs
2	eggs, lightly beaten
2	tablespoons finely chopped fresh mint
¼	teaspoon salt
¼	teaspoon pepper

For sautéing:

½	cup flour
½	cup olive oil

Peel and cut the potato in wedges, place in a small pot, cover with water and simmer for 15 minutes until the potatoes are tender. Drain, transfer to a medium size bowl and mash lightly using a fork.

Grate the zucchini and squeeze out all the moisture with your hands. In a large bowl, combine the zucchini, mashed potato, breadcrumbs, Feta cheese, mint, parsley, salt, pepper and eggs. Mix all the ingredients well and shape into small patties. Flatten slightly and flour both sides.

In a large skillet, heat the olive oil and sauté the zucchini patties on both sides until golden, 1-2 minutes on each side. Serves 6

Stuffed Grape Leaves

1	cup white converted rice
3	cups water
½	cup fresh squeezed lemon juice
1	teaspoon salt
½	cup olive oil
2	cups finely chopped fresh tomatoes
1	cup finely chopped parsley
1	cup finely chopped green onion
½	cup finely chopped fresh mint
½	cup finely chopped fresh dill
¼	teaspoon black pepper
1	16-ounce jar grape leaves
2	cups water

Preheat oven to 350 degrees Fahrenheit.
In a medium size saucepan, cook the rice in 3 cups of water over low heat for 30 minutes. (Do not use minute rice)

In a large bowl combine the cooked rice, olive oil, tomatoes, parsley, onions, mint, dill, salt, pepper, and mix until all the ingredients are blended.

Remove grape leaves from jar and rinse the leaves under cold running water. (the leaves should be bright green, if they are too dark, they have been in the jar too long and will be bitter and tough)

Take one grape leaf at a time, with the vein of the leaf on top, and place 1 tablespoon of the filling in the front-center of the leaf. Fold the top part of the leaf over the rice, while folding the sides, rolling it up like an egg roll. Place the stuffed leaves in a 3-inch deep baking pan and repeat the process until all the rice mixture has been used.

Line the stuffed grape leaves close together to prevent un-folding during baking. Cover the top with one layer of plain leaves to prevent the stuffed grape leaves from browning. Pour the water and lemon juice on top and cover tightly with foil. Bake for 3 hours. Serves 8-10

Yogurt & Cucumber Sauce

2	cups thick yogurt, made from live cultures
1	small European cucumber
4	cloves crushed garlic
1	tablespoon extra olive oil
½	teaspoon hot sauce
	dash of salt

Peel cucumbers and place a grater in a strainer over the sink. Using the large perforated section of the grater, grate the cucumber. Squeeze the grated cucumber against the bottom of the strainer with your hands to remove excess water.

In medium size bowl combine the yogurt with the cucumber, garlic, olive oil, hot sauce and salt. Mix well and refrigerate for two hours before serving. This is a good sauce to enhance the flavor of roasted meat or chicken. Serves 8

Yellow Split Pea Spread

¼	cup olive oil
1	cup chopped yellow onion
5	cups water
1	cup of yellow dried split peas
1	teaspoon salt
¼	teaspoon white ground pepper

For garnish:

½	cup finely sliced red onions
¼	cup finely chopped Italian parsley
1	lemon

In a heavy-bottom medium saucepot, heat the olive oil over medium heat and sauté the onions. Add the water and bring to a boil; add the peas, salt, pepper, and reduce heat to simmer.

Cook for 2½ hours stirring occasionally to prevent sticking to the bottom of the pot. Additional water may be necessary until the peas cook to a soft mashing consistency.

Pour into a shallow serving dish and cool for 2-3 hours before serving. Garnish the top with chopped onions, parsley and freshly squeezed lemon juice. Serve with crusty bread slices. Serves 6

Red Roasted Peppers Stuffed with Goat's Cheese

1	16-ounce jar red roasted peppers
¼	lb goat's cheese
¼	lb Feta cheese, crumbled
2	green onions, finely chopped
2	tablespoons finely chopped fresh red pepper
1	tablespoon finely chopped parsley
1	teaspoon hot sauce

For sautéing:

2	tablespoons olive oil
2	tablespoons flour
1	tablespoon balsamic vinegar
1	tablespoon finely chopped green onions
1	tablespoon finely chopped parsley

In a small bowl combine the Feta, goat's cheese, onions, chopped pepper, hot sauce, parsley, and mix until all the ingredients are well blended.

Remove the roasted peppers from the jar and drain well. Use your hands to gently tear the pepper from the one side to open. Fill the one side of the pepper with a tablespoon of the cheese mixture and fold the empty side to cover the cheese filling. Continue until all the peppers have been stuffed.

Place flour in a large dish and lightly flour each stuffed pepper on both sides, dusting off the excess flour.

In a large frying pan, heat the olive oil over medium heat and sauté the stuffed peppers for one minute on each side. Add the vinegar and chopped green onions to the pan just before removing from heat, sautéing only for about 15 seconds. Serve with toasted pita. Serves 6

Cheese Spread with Smoked Salmon

2	ounces fresh goat's cheese
8	ounces Fata cheese
1	tablespoon finely chopped Kalamata olives
1	tablespoon finely chopped parsley
2	tablespoons finely chopped red onion
1	tablespoon finely chopped red bell pepper
1	teaspoon hot sauce
2	tablespoons pine nuts
8	ounces smoked salmon filet
1	thin banquette loaf, cut in to 24 thin slices

In a small bowl combine the cheeses, olives, parsley, onion, pepper, hot sauce and pine nuts. Mix well to blend the ingredients.

Slice the smoked salmon in 1-inch strips and roll each piece into a coned shape.

Spread a teaspoon of the cheese mixture on each slice of bread and place one piece of rolled salmon on top. Makes 24 pieces. Serves 8

CHAPTER 9

Vegetarian Dishes

Extra virgin olive oil is the cold press oil from superior quality olives and has less than 1% acidity. It is obtained by mechanical and physical methods under controlled conditions; thus, preserving the fruity flavor, color and natural properties of the olive, which contributes to its delicate taste and clear dark green color. Crete, Greece produces the finest olive oil in the world and received the 2002 Mario Solinas Golden Award for the "World's Best Olive Oil" from the International Olive Oil Council, a UN agency based in Madrid. The awarded olive oil was produced in Sitia, Crete.

Pita Pocket Stuffed with Avocado Salad

2	medium avocados
1	tablespoon of fresh squeezed lemon juice
1	ripe tomato, finely chopped
½	cup finely chopped green onion
2	cloves garlic, peeled and finely chopped
1	mild Chile pepper, finely chopped
2	tablespoons finely chopped parsley
2	ounces feta cheese, crumbled
2	large whole-wheat pitas, pocket style
1	tablespoon extra virgin olive oil

Peel and remove the seeds from the avocados, chop in to small pieces and place in a medium bowl with the lemon juice. Toss gently to coat the avocado with the lemon juice.

Add the chopped tomato, onion, garlic, pepper, parsley, feta cheese and olive oil. Mix to blend the ingredients evenly.

Cut the pita pockets in half and toast lightly. Fill each pita half with ¼ of the avocado salad and serve. Serves 4

Portabella Mushroom Sandwiches

2	*tablespoons extra virgin olive oil*
1	*large Portabella mushroom, sliced*
½	*red bell pepper, sliced into rings*
6	*medium red onion rings*
	salt to taste
1	*tablespoon balsamic vinegar*
1	*ounce white cheddar cheese*
½	*avocado, sliced*
2	*small whole-wheat buns*

In a large frying pan, heat the olive oil over low heat and sauté the mushroom slices, onions and pepper rings until lightly golden. Salt lightly to taste, and finish with a tablespoon of balsamic vinegar.

Toast the whole-wheat buns and arrange the sautéed mushroom slices on the half portion of each bun, dividing equally between the two buns.

Add the grated cheese and pile the onions, peppers and avocado slices on top, followed by the other half of the wheat bun. Serves 2

Note: This sandwich makes up two of the bread servings for the day.

Black-eyed Peas with Rice

1	10-ounce package frozen black-eyed peas
¼	cup extra virgin olive oil
¼	cup finely chopped green onion
2	tablespoons finely chopped fresh parsley
2	tablespoons finely chopped fresh mint
½	teaspoon salt
	dash of black pepper
2	cups water
½	cup white converted rice

Defrost the black-eyed peas.

In a medium size saucepan, heat the olive oil and sauté the onions until they are translucent.

Add the black-eyed peas, parsley, mint, salt, pepper and water.

When the water starts simmering, add the rice and cook for 30 minutes. Serves 6

Green Beans with Tomatoes and Herbs

1	lb fresh green beans
½	cup finely chopped onion
¼	cup extra virgin olive oil
½	teaspoon sugar
1	lb ripe red tomatoes
1	cup water
1	tablespoon finely chopped fresh dill
2	cloves garlic, minced
2	tablespoons chopped Italian parsley
½	teaspoon salt
	dash of allspice

Trim the ends off the green beans, cut in half, place in a strainer and rinse under cold water.

Grate or crush the tomatoes into a small bowl and set aside.

In a medium pot, heat the olive oil and sauté the onions with the sugar, stirring until they become translucent.

Add the crushed tomatoes, parsley, dill, garlic, allspice, salt and water. Simmer for 2-3 minutes, add the green beans and cook for 30 minutes longer or until the green beans become tender.

The cooking time depends on the freshness of the green beans. Serves 6

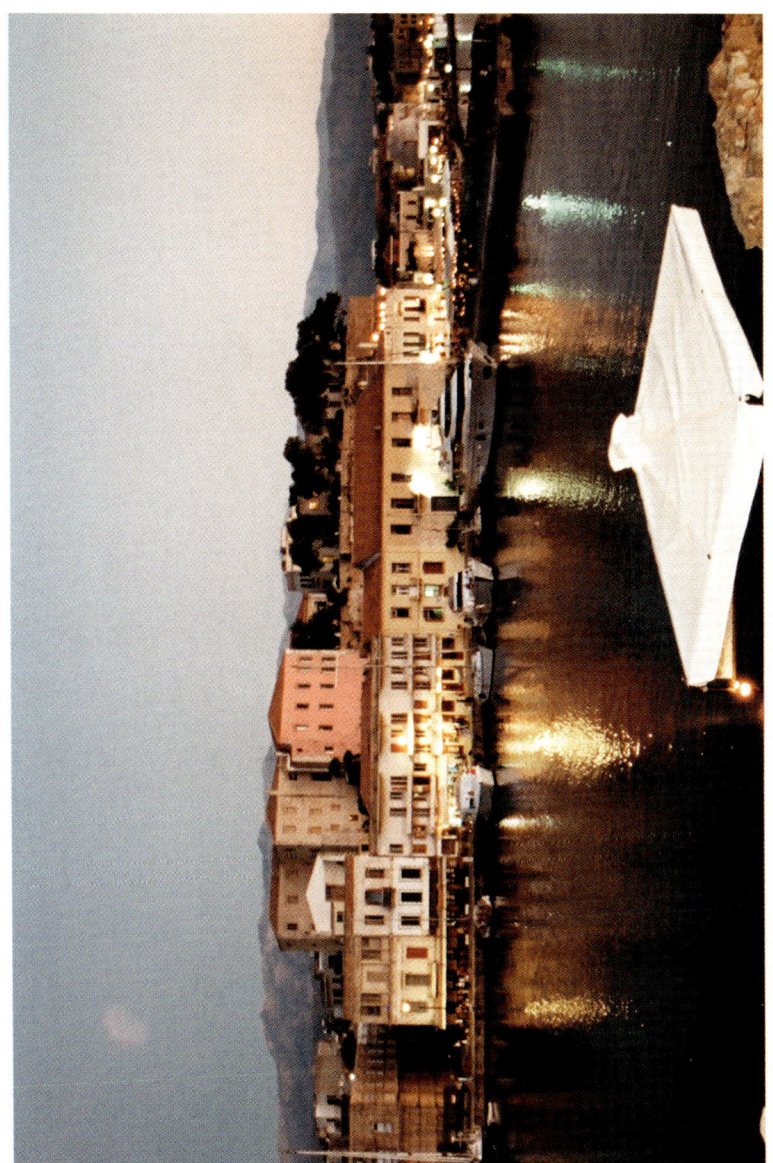
Hania, Crete

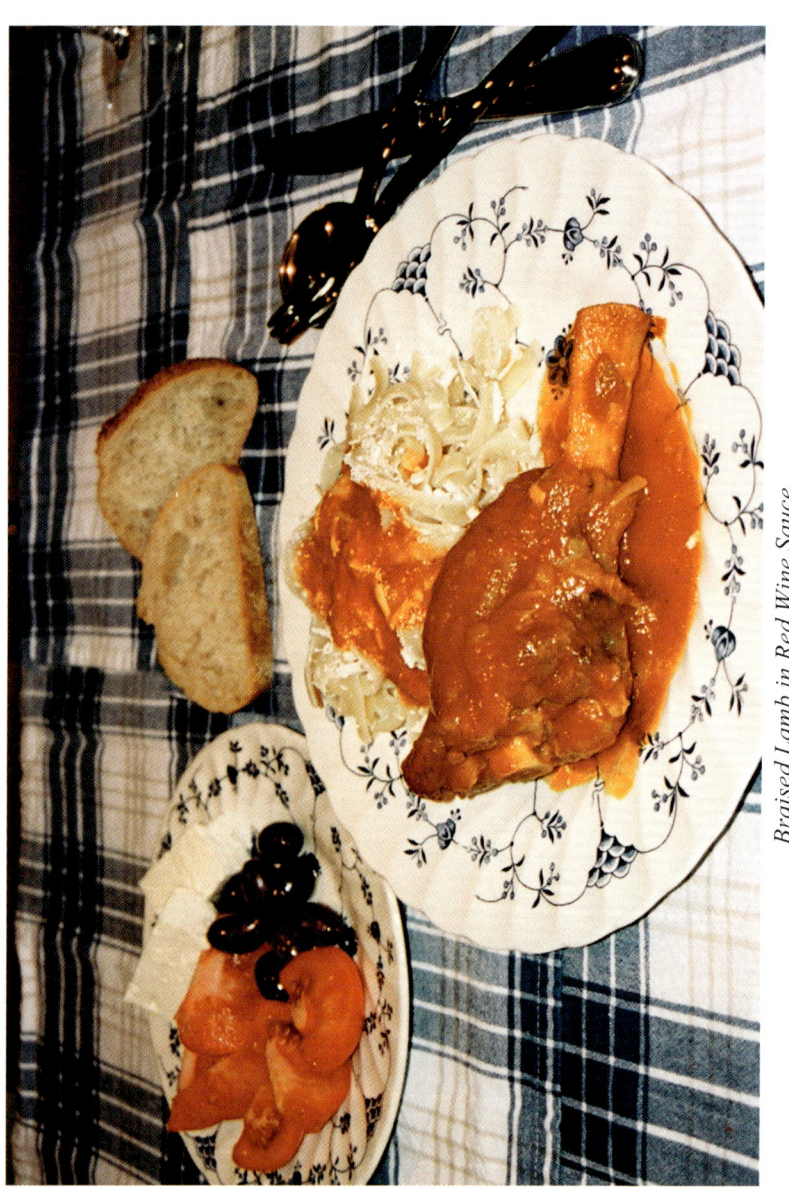

Braised Lamb in Red Wine Sauce

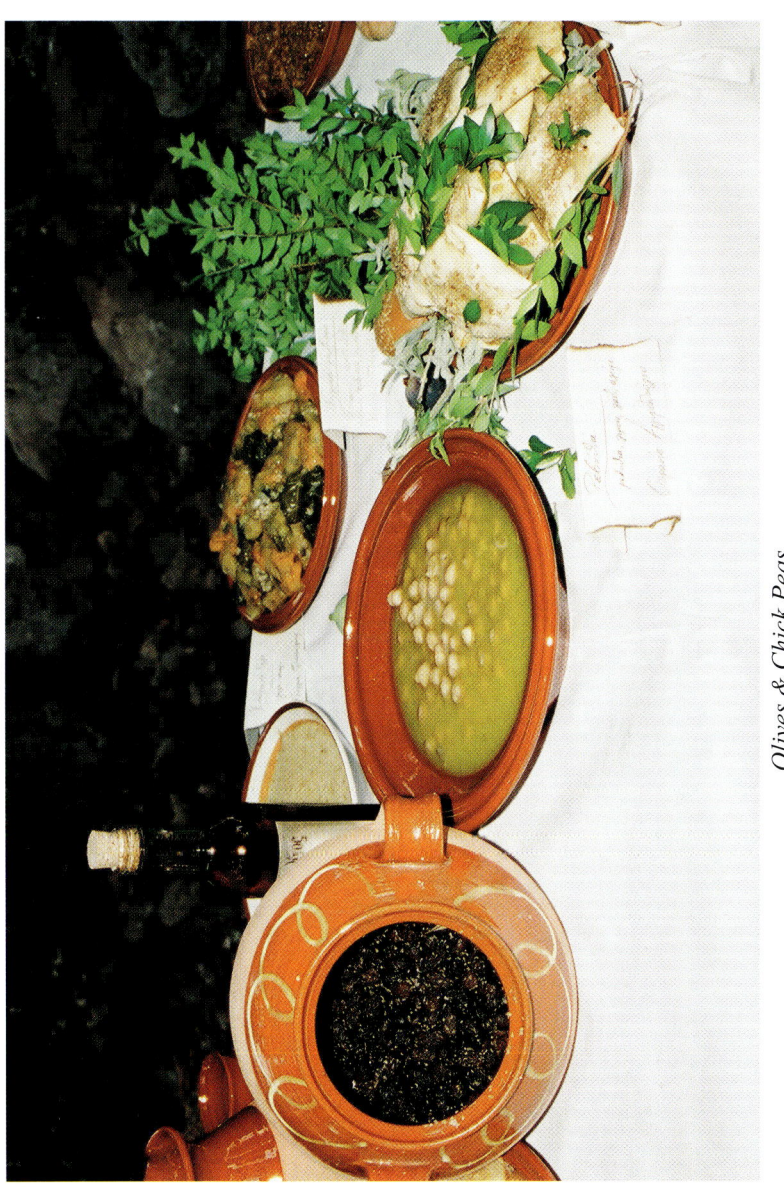

Olives & Chick Peas

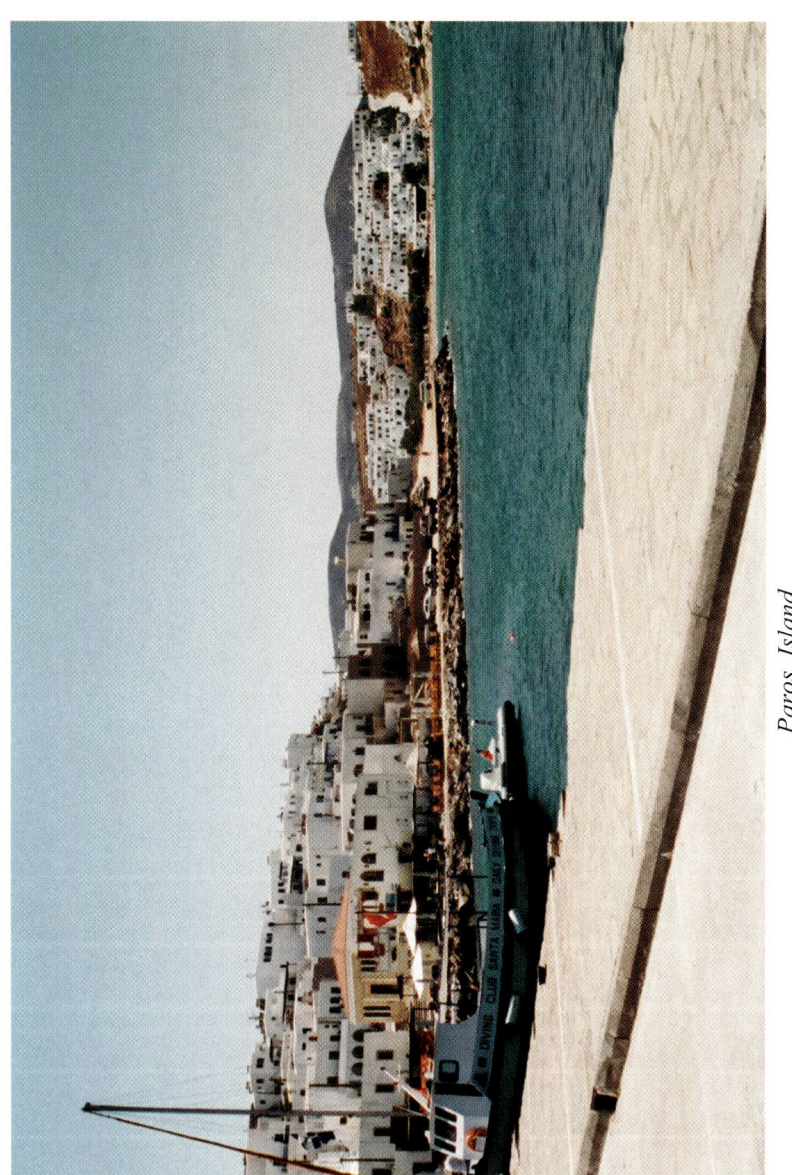

Paros, Island

Fettuccine with Garlic & Basil

6	cloves garlic, crushed
6	tablespoons olive oil
1	lb fresh Roma tomatoes, finely chopped
1	lb Fettuccine pasta
1	ounce finely chopped basil
½	cup pine nuts
4	ounces Romano cheese, grated

Fill a large pot with 4 quarts water and a tablespoon of salt. Bring the water to boil, add the pasta and cook for 15-20 to el dente (tender but firm). Cooking time depends on the brand, therefore, follow the package directions and do not overcook! Drain, and prepare the remaining ingredients.

In a large skillet, heat the olive oil over medium heat, sear the garlic lightly and add the chopped tomatoes. Add the cooked pasta to the skillet and using tongs, toss to coat the pasta with the olive oil. Remove from heat and add the basil, pine nuts and cheese, tossing to combine all the ingredients evenly. Transfer to a serving platter. Serves 8

Risotto with Spinach

2	cups chicken stock
½	cup risotto
½	teaspoon salt
1	lb fresh spinach, leaves only
1	cup chopped green onion
¼	cup extra virgin olive oil
1	oz fresh dill, chopped

In a medium saucepan, heat the stock over low heat and bring to a simmer. Add the risotto and salt. Continue to simmer on low heat for 25-30 minutes until all the moisture is absorbed. Remove from heat and set aside.

In another saucepan, heat the olive oil over medium heat and sauté the onions and spinach leaves lightly until they become wilted.

Add the risotto and dill to the spinach and stir with a large spoon to mix all the ingredients. Cook for 3 to 5 minutes over low heat until all the moisture from the spinach is absorbed. Serves 6

Artichokes with Potatoes, Dill & Lemon

3	fresh artichokes or one pound frozen
¼	cup extra virgin olive oil
½	cup chopped green onion
1	cup baby carrots
½	cup chopped dill
1	cup water
1	lb white or red potatoes
1	teaspoon salt
¼	teaspoon pepper
1	cup fresh squeezed lemon juice

Peel and clean the artichoke hearts by removing the hard outer leaves and fuzzy portion in the center.

Cut artichoke hearts in 4 quarters and soak them in cold water mixed with half of the lemon juice. (This will prevent oxidation from exposure to the air, which causes browning).

Peel and cut the potatoes in half, and drain the artichokes.

In a medium sauce pan heat oil and sauté the onions with the artichokes for 2 minutes. Add 1 cup water, potatoes, carrots, dill, salt, pepper and the remaining lemon juice.

Cook over medium heat until the liquid starts to boil. Lower the heat and simmer for 30 minutes. Serves 6

Garlic Mashed Potatoes

2	lbs bake style potatoes
4	cloves garlic, crushed
4	tablespoons extra virgin olive oil
¼	cup warm milk
½	teaspoon salt

Peel and cut potatoes into wedges, place them in a medium saucepan and cover with water. Cook over medium heat until the potatoes are tender (15-20 minutes). Do not overcook.

Drain and transfer into a mixing bowl.

Using an electric mixer beat the potatoes on low speed for one minute; add the garlic, olive oil, milk and salt. Beat two minutes until well blended and smooth. Serves 6

Baked Beans

1	lb dried lima beans
1	rounded teaspoon salt
½	cup extra virgin olive oil
1	cup chopped onion
½	cup chopped parsley
2	cups crushed tomatoes
2	bay leaves
2	cloves garlic, sliced
2	mild green Chile peppers, whole

Soak the lima beans for eight hours in two quarts of cold water. The beans should double in size.

Drain and place in an ovenproof pot. Add two quarts of water, the salt, and bring to a boil. Reduce the heat and simmer for 2 hours, stirring occasionally.

Preheat oven to 350 degrees Fahrenheit. In a large skillet sauté the onions in olive oil until golden.

After the beans have simmered for 2 hours, add the sautéed onions, parsley, tomatoes, bay leaves, garlic and peppers. Bake in a preheated oven for 1 hour. Serves 8-10

Seared Vegetables

4	tablespoons extra virgin olive oil
1	small yellow bell pepper, sliced
1	small red bell pepper, sliced
1	medium onion, peeled and sliced
1	yellow squash
½	lb fresh asparagus
½	cup baby carrots
4	cloves garlic, sliced
½	ounce fresh oregano, finely chopped
	salt and pepper to taste

Remove the hard stems off the asparagus, cut in half and prepare the remaining vegetables. Heat olive oil in a large skillet or Wok and sauté the vegetables and garlic for 5 minutes, tossing continually. Add the fresh oregano, salt and pepper, and stir. Serve with pita bread. Serves 6

Rice Pilaf

3	cups chicken stock
1	teaspoon of salt
1	cup white converted rice

In a 4-quart sauce-pan combine stock, salt, and bring to a boil over medium heat. Reduce heat to low, add the rice and simmer for 30 minutes. Serves 6

Steamed Greens

1	lb kale
1	lb mustard greens
4	tablespoons olive oil
¼	teaspoon salt
2	cloves garlic
½	lb mushrooms, sliced
1	lemon
4	ounces Feta cheese, crumbled

Trim off the tough stems from the kale and mustard greens, cut the leaves in half and wash in the sink to remove all the dirt. Drain.

In a large pot bring 1-cup of water to boil and add the greens. Steam for 5-10 minutes until all greens are slightly wilted. Drain in a colander for one minute and transfer to a serving platter.

In a large skillet, heat the olive oil and sauté the mushrooms and garlic for 2 minutes over medium heat. Squeeze lemon juice over the spinach and spoon the mushrooms, crumbled feta cheese, garlic and olive oil over the top. Serve with garlic toast. Serves 4

Eggplant Vinaigrette

2	lbs small Japanese eggplant
¼	cup extra virgin olive oil
1	medium onion, peeled and sliced thin
4	cloves garlic, sliced thin
2	tablespoons tomato paste diluted in 1-cup water
1	tablespoon fresh oregano, chopped
2	tablespoons finely chopped parsley
½	teaspoon salt
1	teaspoon pepper
2	tablespoons balsamic vinegar

Preheat oven to 400 degrees Fahrenheit.
Cut the stems off the eggplant, slice in half, lengthwise, and season with salt.

Place the sliced eggplant in a large bowl; add enough water to cover and place a heavy plate on top to hold the eggplant submersed in water for 15 minutes (this process removes the bitterness). Drain and dry the eggplant slices on a paper towel.

In a large sauce pot, heat the olive oil and sear the onions and garlic over medium heat until golden. Add the tomato paste diluted in water and bring to simmer. Add eggplant, oregano, parsley, vinegar, salt and pepper, and simmer for 5 minutes.

Transfer into a baking dish and bake in a preheated oven for 20 minutes. Serves 6

Spinach with Red Peppers & Almonds

1	lb spinach, leaves only
1	red bell pepper, sliced
½	cup sliced almonds
¼	cup extra virgin olive oil
1	fresh lemon
4	cloves garlic, sliced
	salt and pepper to taste
3	lb fresh goat's cheese

Place spinach in a large pot filled with cold water and rinse and drain well.

Place the spinach in a large pot with ½ cup water over low heat and steam until the spinach has wilted (2-3 minutes). Drain in a colander and transfer to a serving platter.

Heat olive oil in a medium saucepot and sauté the peppers, almonds and garlic for 2-3 minutes until slightly golden.

Spoon the olive oil contents over the spinach, season with salt and pepper, and squeeze fresh lemon juice on top. Serve each portion with ½-once of goat's cheese and a slice of toasted French bread. Serves 6

Tomatoes Stuffed with Rice & Herbs

6	medium size ripe tomatoes
½	cup chopped green pepper
1	small zucchini, finely chopped
6	small potatoes
¼	cup extra virgin olive oil
½	cup finely chopped onion
3	large cloves garlic, finely chopped
½	cup finely chopped Italian parsley
¼	cup finely chopped fresh mint
1	cup white converted rice
1	cup water
½	teaspoon salt
¼	teaspoon pepper

For the sauce:

2	cups water
6	ounces tomato paste
2	tablespoons extra virgin olive oil
½	teaspoon Greek oregano
½	teaspoon salt
¼	teaspoon pepper

Preheat oven to 350 degrees Fahrenheit.
Slice the tops of the tomatoes off to allow an opening of two inches wide. Using a small spoon, remove the inner pulp from the tomatoes and set aside.

Peel and cut the potatoes in half and chop the onions, zucchini, pepper and tomato pulp into small pieces.

In a large skillet heat the olive oil and sauté the chopped vegetables for 2-3 minutes on medium heat. Add the rice, water, mint, garlic parsley, salt and pepper. Simmer for 20 minutes until the water is absorbed.

Using a small spoon fill the hollow tomatoes with the rice stuffing and cover with the previously sliced tomato-tops. Place the stuffed tomatoes in a 13X11X2 inch pan and arrange the potatoes in between.

To prepare the sauce, dilute the tomato paste in the water and add the olive oil, oregano, salt and pepper. Mix well and pour over the tomatoes and potatoes. Cover with aluminum foil and bake for 45 minutes, uncover and bake 30 minutes longer. Serves 6

Spinach & Cheese Pie

1 ¼   lbs spinach, leaves only
¼   cup olive oil
1   cup chopped green onions
¼   lb leaks, chopped
1   lb feta cheese, crumbled
2   ounces fresh dill, chopped
4   eggs, lightly beaten
¼   teaspoon salt
2   tablespoons flour

For the pastry:

1/3   cup extra virgin olive oil, slightly warmed
½   lb phyllo pastry dough

Defrost the pastry in the refrigerator overnight, and preheat oven to 350 degrees Fahrenheit, before you begin preparation.

Wash the spinach, green onions and leaks in a kitchen sink or a large bowl filled with cold water. Rinse several times to remove all the dirt and drain in a colander.

Remove all excess water by squeezing the spinach leaves with your hands against the bottom of the colander.

In a small saucepan, heat the olive oil over medium heat and sauté the onions and leaks for 3 minutes.

In a large bowl combine the spinach, onions and leaks, dill, salt, eggs, flour and Feta cheese. Mix well with hands and set aside.

Unfold phyllo pastry gently and using a pastry brush, coat the bottom and sides of the pan with the olive oil.

Place eight to ten layers of the pastry on the bottom of the pan, one piece of the pastry at a time, brushing each leaf lightly with the olive oil, allowing four of the layers to extend two inches over the sides of the pan.

Pour the spinach mixture into the pan and spread evenly. Fold in the pastry that extends to the side and layer the remaining pastry on top, brushing each piece lightly with olive oil. Tuck in the edges with the pastry brush for a neat presentation.

With a sharp knife cut the top layer gently all the way to the bottom (two rows lengthwise and three rows and then tree rows the opposite direction), dividing the pie into six square pieces. Cut each piece on an angle (corner to corner) in two triangular pieces.

Bake for 1 hour, until golden. Serve hot or cold. Serves 12

Potatoes with Green Peas

6	tablespoons olive oil
1	medium white onion, peeled and chopped
1	clove peeled garlic
½	cup crushed ripe tomatoes
2	cups water
2	lbs potatoes, peeled and cut in quarters
1	lb frozen petite green peas
2	tablespoons freshly chopped parsley
½	ounce fresh dill, chopped
½	teaspoon salt
	dash of pepper

In a medium size pot, heat the olive oil and sauté the onions with the garlic.

Add the tomatoes and sauté 1 minute, add the water and bring the sauce to a simmer over low heat. Add the potatoes, peas, salt and pepper, and simmer in a covered saucepan for 25 minutes.

Add the dill and parsley, and cook for 5 minutes longer. Serves 5-6. May be served hot or cold.

Potatoes with Oregano & Lemon

4	Russet potatoes, peeled and cut in quarters
¼	cup extra virgin olive oil
¼	teaspoon oregano
2	cloves garlic, sliced
1	cup chicken stock or water
¼	teaspoon salt
	juice of one lemon and pepper to taste

Preheat oven to 375 degrees Fahrenheit. In a large bowl combine all the ingredients and mix well with hands. Transfer to a 10X13 inch-roasting pan, cover and bake for 1 hour. Uncover and bake for 30 minutes longer until the potatoes turn golden. Serves 4

Butter Beans with Dill

2	10-ounce packages frozen butter beans
4	tablespoons olive oil
½	cup chopped white onion
½	cup chopped green onion
½	ounce fresh dill, finely chopped
2	cups chicken stock
½	teaspoon salt

Defrost beans. In a medium saucepan heat the olive oil and cook the onions until they are soft and translucent. Add the beans, dill, stock and salt. Stir, cover, and simmer over low heat for 30 minutes. Serves 6

Chapter 10

Meat & Poultry Dishes

Sitia, Crete

Sitia is a small city on the northeast coastline of Crete, covered in vineyards, and meadows with bananas and apple trees. The view from the mountains is unforgettable! The blue sky appears endless with beautiful peninsulas stretching into the deep blue sea, with little cafés close to the shore serving the best fresh seafood. This is the place where my mother was born, and the birthplace of many famous artists and poets. Just a few miles outside Sitia, to the far-east coast, there is a palm-tree forest called "Vai," which appears to be untouched by civilization. Its white sandy beaches make you feel as though you are the only person to step into the sand, and you become mesmerized as you watch the Sun climb up from the endless blue sea.

Lamb Chops with Mushrooms & Mint

6	lamb chops (4 ounces each)
½	lb mushrooms, sliced
2	cloves garlic, finely chopped
¼	cup finely chopped onion
¼	cup olive oil
2	tablespoons finely chopped mint
	salt and pepper to taste
1	tablespoon flour
1	cup red wine

Trim the fat off the lamb chops, season with salt and pepper and lightly flour.

In a large skillet, heat the olive oil and sauté the lamb chops for 2 minutes on each side.

Transfer the lamp chops to a plate. In the same skillet add the mushrooms, garlic, onions and mint and sauté for 2 minutes over medium heat.

Return the chops to the skillet, add the wine and cook for 2 additional minutes until the sauce thickens. Serve 1 chop per person with two tablespoons of mushroom sauce. Serves 6

Braised Lamb in Red Wine Sauce

2	lbs boneless leg of lamb (or six small shoulder chops or shanks)
¼	cup olive oil
½	cup finely chopped onions
12	ounces tomato paste
6	cups water
1	teaspoon salt
½	teaspoon pepper
1	stick cinnamon
1	clove garlic, peeled and sliced
½	cup red wine
1	lb linguine pasta
4	ounces grated Myzithra or Parmesan cheese

Trim all the visible fat off the lamb and cut in six equal portions or use 6 small lamb shanks. In a large heavy-bottom braising pot, heat the olive oil over medium heat and brown the lamb with the onions.

Add the tomato paste diluted in the water, garlic, cinnamon stick, salt and pepper. Braise for 2 hours on low heat, turning the meat at least twice during cooking. Remove the cinnamon stick, add the wine and cook another 15 minutes.

Cook the pasta according to package directions. Add the grated cheese on the cooked pasta and toss. Serve a portion of lamb with 1 cup of pasta and ¼ cup of the sauce. Serves 6-8

Lamb with Pine Nuts & Raisins

2	lbs boneless leg of lamb
4	tablespoons olive oil
½	cup finely chopped onion
1	teaspoon salt
¼	teaspoon freshly ground pepper
2	cups water
½	cup orange juice
½	teaspoon coriander
½	teaspoon nutmeg
1	cup white converted rice
1	tablespoon grated orange rind
½	cup white raisins
1	cup pine nuts

Trim all the visible fat from the lamb, cut in small pieces, and season with salt and pepper.

Heat the olive oil over medium heat and sear the meat with the onions until golden.

Add the water, juice, spices, and cook over low heat for one hour.

Add the rice and simmer for 20 minutes; add the orange rind, pine nuts and raisins and cook 5 minutes longer. Serves 6-8

Roasted Lamb & Potatoes

2	lbs boneless leg of lamb
½	teaspoon salt
¼	teaspoon pepper
¼	cup wine
6	medium baked potatoes
¼	cup fresh squeezed lemon juice
3	cloves garlic, peeled and sliced
1	teaspoon oregano
3	tablespoons olive oil
½	teaspoon salt
¼	teaspoon freshly ground pepper

Preheat oven to 400 degrees Fahrenheit. Season the lamb with salt, pepper and half the oregano.

Place in a deep roasting pan (15"X13") and roast in the preheated oven for 30 minutes.

Meanwhile, peel and cut the potatoes in wedges. In a large bowl combine potatoes, lemon juice, olive oil, garlic, remaining oregano, salt and pepper, and mix well with hands.

Pour the wine on top of the roast and arrange the potatoes around it. Continue roasting for 1 hour longer or until potatoes are tender.

Remove from oven and let the lamb roast stand 10 minutes before slicing. Place the meat on a cutting board and carve into slices. Serves 6

Pork Tenderloin with Apples & Apricots

2	lbs pork tenderloin
4	tablespoons olive oil
½	cup finely chopped fresh green onion
2	apples
4	ripe apricots
2	cups chicken stock
2	tablespoons finely chopped fresh thyme
1	teaspoon of salt
¼	teaspoon white pepper
½	cup white wine
¼	cup flour

Rinse the meat under cold water and remove the visible fat and transparent skin. Cut the pork into 1-inch thick round pieces approximately two ounces each. Season with salt, white pepper and lightly flour.

Peel and core the apples, wash the apricots and remove the pits. Cut the fruit in thin slices and set aside.

In a large skillet heat the olive oil and sear each side of the pork for 1 minute with the onions. Add the apples, apricots, chicken stock, wine and thyme. Cover and simmer for 10 minutes on low heat. Serve two pieces of meat with two tablespoons of fruit per serving portions. Serves 8

Baked Italian Meatballs

2	lbs extra lean ground beef (>90% lean)
¼	cup plain breadcrumbs
1	medium onion, grated
¼	cup low-fat milk
1	egg
2	tablespoons finely chopped parsley
½	cup finely chopped fresh basil
½	teaspoon salt
¼	teaspoon pepper
¼	teaspoon nutmeg

For The Tomato Sauce:

½	cup olive oil
½	cup finely chopped onion
3	cloves garlic, finely chopped
1	12-ounce canned tomato paste diluted in
6	cups water
½	teaspoon salt
1	teaspoon dried Greek oregano
½	cup red wine

Preheat oven to 375 degrees Fahrenheit.
Place the ground beef in a large mixing bowl and break the meat apart with your hands; add the breadcrumbs, grated onion, milk, egg, parsley, basil, salt, pepper and nutmeg. Mix well with hands until all the ingredients are blended well. Pinch off a small portion of meat and shape it into

a meatball (should make approximately 24). Place the meatballs in a shallow baking pan and bake in the preheated oven for 30 minutes.

Meanwhile, sauté the onions in the olive oil over medium heat; add the tomato paste diluted in the water, garlic, oregano, salt and wine. Simmer for 10 minutes over low heat. Add the baked meatballs to the sauce and simmer for 20 minutes on low heat. Serve with pasta or plain. Serves 8

Veal Scaloppini

4	4-ounce pieces veal cutlets
2	tablespoons flour
2	tablespoons extra virgin olive oil
2	tablespoons finely chopped chives
1	tablespoon finely chopped fresh sage
2	tablespoons small capers
1	cup chicken stock
¼	cup white wine
	salt and pepper to taste

Flatten each piece of veal using the flat side of a mallet, and season with salt and pepper. Coat lightly with the flour and dust off the excess.

Heat the olive oil in a large skillet and sauté the veal for 1 minute on each side, add the wine, stock, and remaining ingredients. Simmer for 3-5 minutes until the sauce thickens. Serve with rice pilaf. Serves 4

Baked Ziti with Meat Sauce

2	lbs extra lean ground beef (>90% lean)
1	cup chopped onions
¼	cup olive oil
¼	teaspoon nutmeg
¼	cup freshly chopped oregano
1	teaspoon of salt
½	teaspoon pepper
2	6-ounce cans tomato paste
4	cups water
¼	cup chopped flat parsley
½	cup wine

For the pasta:

1	lb Ziti pasta
2	quarts water
1	teaspoon of salt
4	ounces grated Parmesan
4	ounces Mozzarella

Preheat oven to 350 degrees Fahrenheit.
In a large sauce pot heat the olive oil and brown the meat with the onions, stirring frequently to break the meat to small pieces during browning.

Add the salt, pepper, tomato paste diluted in the water, oregano, parsley and nutmeg. Stir until the ingredients are mixed well and simmer for 30 minutes, add the wine and cook for 5 more minutes.

In a large pot bring 2 quarts of water to boil, add the pasta and 1 teaspoon of salt. Cook for 12 minutes and drain. Pour pasta into baking pan (13X11X2"), add the grated cheese and spread the pasta evenly across the pan. Use a ladle to pour the hot meat sauce over and in-between the pasta.

Sprinkle grated Mozzarella on top and bake in a preheated oven for 15 minutes. Serves 8-10

Spanish Salsa

4	tomatoes, finely chopped
¼	cup finely chopped cilantro
1	large avocado, finely chopped
½	cup finely chopped onion
2	mild green Chiles, finely chopped
4	tablespoons olive oil
½	teaspoon dried Greek oregano
	salt and pepper to taste

In a medium size bowl combine all the ingredients and mix well. Marinate for 1 hour before serving.

Serve as an appetizer with pita or as an accompaniment to Enchiladas and Burritos.

Chicken Enchiladas

1	lb chicken breast
1	16-ounces Enchilada sauce
8	medium flour tortillas
3	tablespoons olive oil
1	cup chopped yellow onions
2	medium ripe tomatoes, chopped
1	cup chopped mild green Chiles
2	tablespoons chopped black olives
12	ounces Monterey Jack and yellow cheddar cheese, grated

Preheat oven to 350 degrees Fahrenheit and cut the chicken breast in very thin strips.

In a large skillet, heat the olive oil and sauté the chicken with the onions until golden. Add the green chilies, olives and tomatoes. Mix well and continue to cook for 5 minutes on low heat.

Pour the enchilada sauce in a large bowl. Take one tortilla at a time and dip it in the enchilada sauce, coating both sides. Place each tortilla on a plate and fill with two heaping tablespoons of the chicken mixture and one ounce of the grated cheese.

Fold the front portion of the tortilla over the top to wrap the chicken mixture and place each wrapped enchilada in a baking pan carefully, with the folded part of the tortilla facing the bottom of the pan.

Repeat with the rest of the tortillas until all the ingredients have been used. Pour the remaining sauce over the enchiladas and sprinkle the remaining grated cheese on top.

Bake in the preheated oven for 15 minutes. Serve with yogurt, chopped lettuce and Spanish salsa. Serves 8

Green Chile Sauce

2	tablespoons extra virgin olive oil
1	cup finely chopped green onion
1	lb fresh green Chile peppers
3	cloves garlic, crushed
3	cups chicken stock
1	tablespoon finely chopped fresh oregano
½	teaspoon salt
	dash of black pepper
2	tablespoons cornstarch diluted in
2	tablespoons water

Remove the seeds and stems from the Chile peppers and chop into small pieces.

In a medium saucepan heat the olive oil over low heat and sauté the onions with the Chile peppers and garlic until slightly wilted. Add the stock, oregano, salt and pepper and bring to boil. Reduce heat and add the cornstarch mixture stirring quickly to thicken. Simmer on the low heat for 30 minutes, stirring occasionally. Makes 3-4 cups.

Beef Burritos with Green Chile Sauce

For the burritos:

4	tortillas
1	lb thinly sliced roast beef
4	ounces cheddar cheese, grated
3	cups Chile Sauce from page 181

Side condiments:

2	cups shredded lettuce
2	cups low-fat yogurt

Preheat the oven to 375 degrees Fahrenheit.
Place 4 ounces of sliced roast beef in the center of each tortilla. Add 1 ounce of grated cheese on top of the beef and ¼ cup green Chile sauce.

Wrap the tortillas and place them on a non-stick baking pan, with the closure toward the bottom of the pan. Pour the remaining sauce on top and bake in the hot oven for 20 minutes to melt the cheese. Serve with shredded lettuce, Spanish salsa and ½ cup of low fat yogurt.

Oriental Chicken & Shrimp

1	lb boneless and skinless chicken breast
½	lb shrimp, peeled and de-veined
4	tablespoons olive oil
½	teaspoon dried ginger
1	cup sliced yellow onions
1	cup baby carrots
1	red bell pepper, sliced thin
½	lb fresh or frozen pea pods
1	cup chicken stock
½	cup unsweetened pineapple juice
1	tablespoon cornstarch
3	tablespoons soy sauce
	salt and pepper to taste

Rinse the chicken and shrimp under cold water and let it dry on a paper towel. Cut the chicken in thin strips and season lightly with salt and pepper.

Heat the olive oil in a large skillet and sear the chicken with the shrimp, onions, peppers, carrots, pea pods and ginger until golden. Using tongs, remove the shrimp from the skillet, add the stock and soy sauce, and continue simmering for another 15 minutes over low heat.

Return the shrimp to the skillet, and add the cornstarch diluted in the pineapple juice, stirring until the sauce thickens. Serve with rice pilaf or oriental noodles. Serves 6

Roasted Chicken & Potatoes

1	3-lb chicken for roasting
3	lbs potatoes
½	teaspoon Greek oregano
4	cloves garlic, sliced
¼	cup olive oil
2	cups water
½	cup lemon juice
1	teaspoon of salt
¼	teaspoon pepper

Preheat oven to 375 degrees Fahrenheit. Remove the skin and fat from the chicken and rinse under cold water.

Peel and cut the potatoes in quarters and place in a large roasting pan with the chicken pieces. Add the water, lemon juice, garlic, oregano, olive oil, salt and pepper, and mix well using a large spoon or clean hands.

Bake in a preheated oven for 1-1/2 hours or until potatoes and chicken are golden and tender. Serves 8

Roasted Cornish Hens with Apples & Raisins

4	Cornish game hens (28 ounces each)
	salt and pepper to taste
1	tablespoon olive oil
1	teaspoon butter
2	cups chopped green apples, cored
½	cup golden raisins
¼	teaspoon ginger
¼	teaspoon thyme
	dash of cinnamon
½	cup white wine
½	cup chicken stock

Heat oven to 425 degrees Fahrenheit. Cut the hens in half, rinse under cold water and season with salt and pepper. Place the hens in a roasting pan and roast for 35 minutes.

In a small saucepot, heat the olive oil and butter over low heat and cook the apples for 2 minutes.

Add raisins, thyme, ginger, cinnamon, stock and wine; continue to simmer for 3 minutes. Spoon the fruit glaze over the hens and bake 15 minutes longer. Serve with rice pilaf. Serves 8

Chicken with Herbs & Wine

1	4 lb whole chicken
½	teaspoon salt
¼	teaspoon pepper
3	tablespoons extra virgin olive oil
2	tablespoons freshly chopped green onions
1	tablespoon freshly chopped marjoram
1	tablespoon freshly chopped thyme
	dash of cayenne pepper
1	tablespoon grated orange rind
½	cup white wine
1	cup chicken stock

Rinse the chicken under cold running water and remove the skin and fat, cut into eight pieces and season with salt and pepper.

In a large skillet, heat the olive oil over medium heat and sauté the chicken on both sides until golden. Add the onions and continue to cook until the onions are translucent.

Add the marjoram, thyme, pepper, orange rind, wine and stock; simmer on low heat for 30 minutes. Serves 8

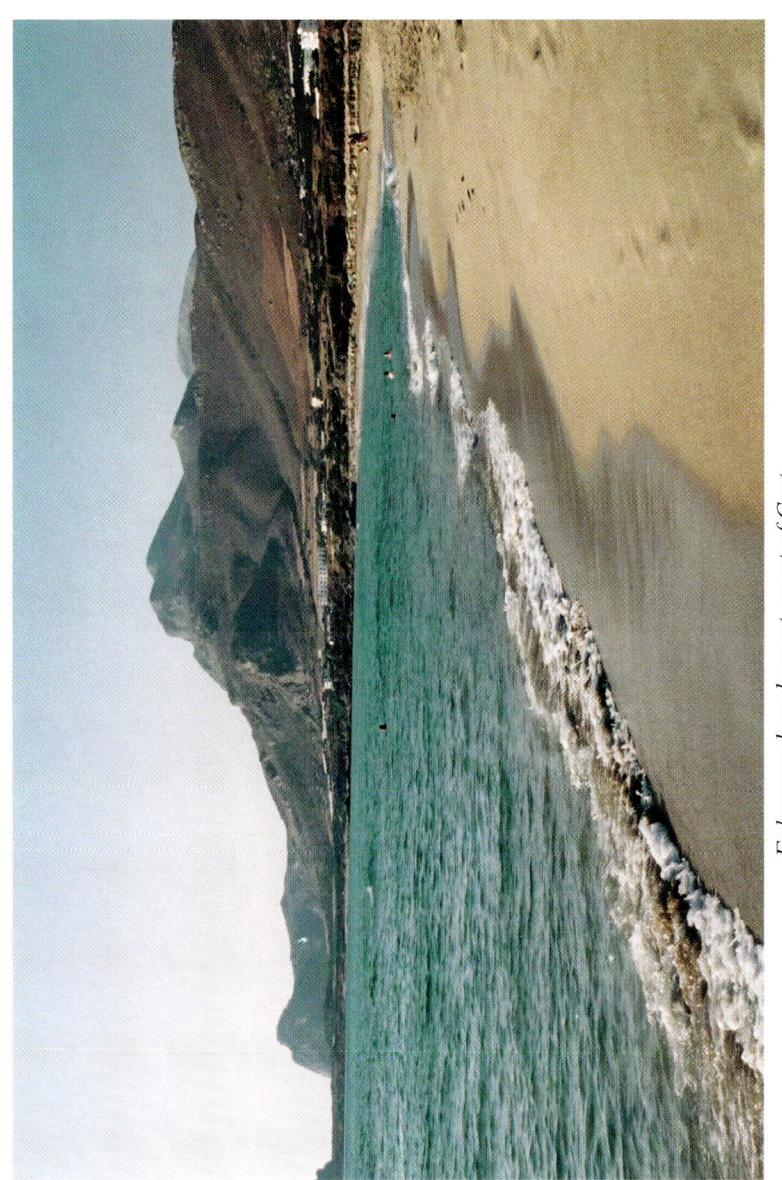

Falaserna beach, west coast of Crete

Grilled Trout

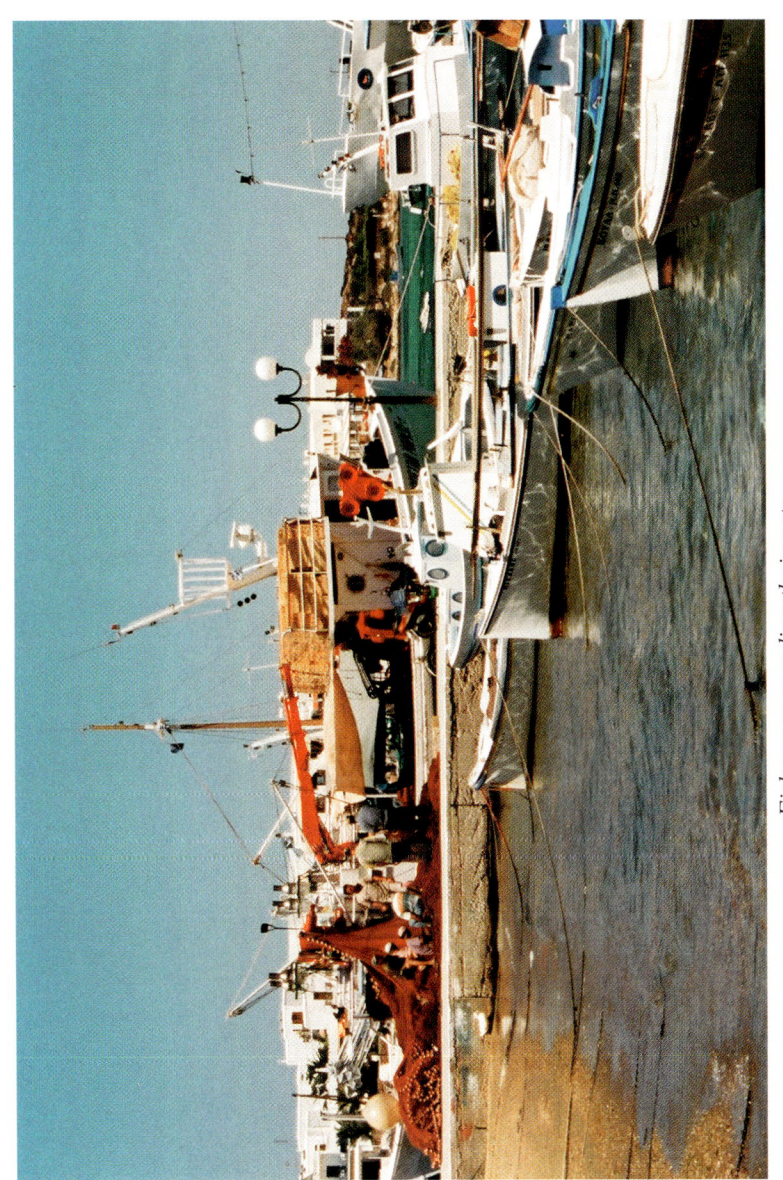

Fishermen mending their nets

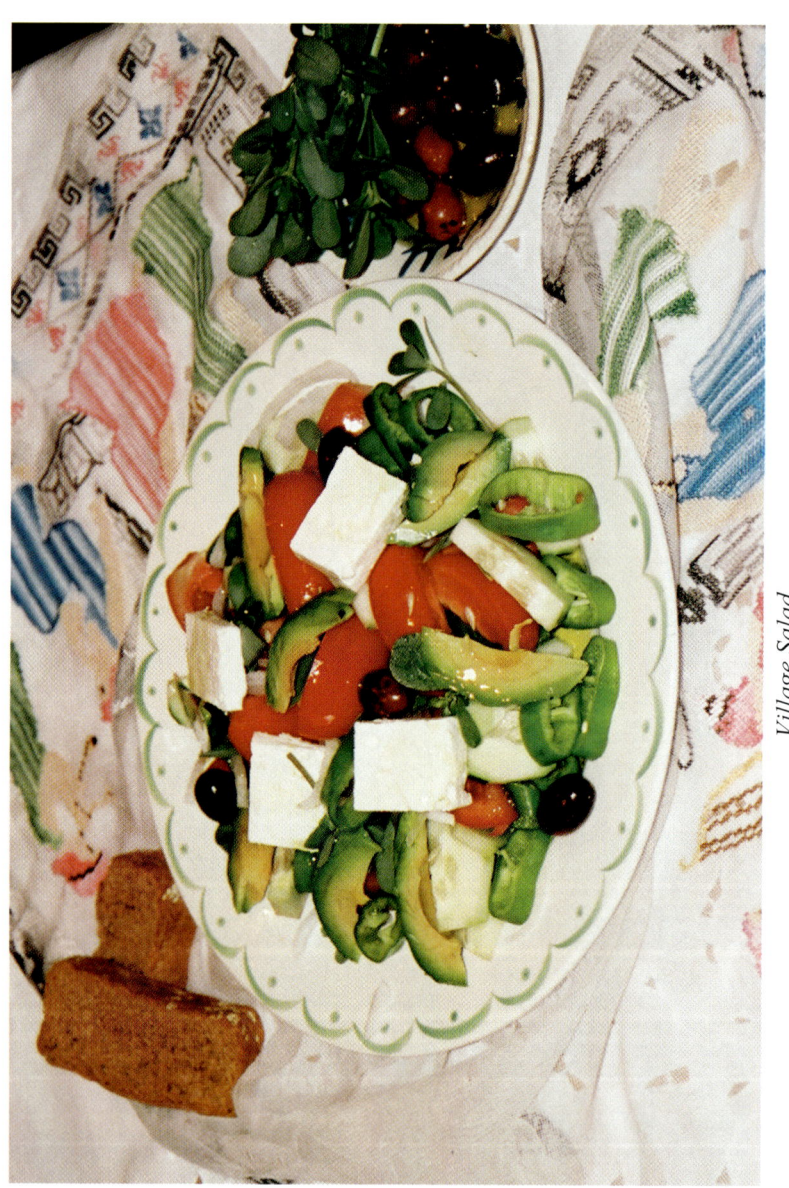

Village Salad

CHAPTER 11

Seafood Dishes

Hania, Crete

The Old Town of Hania has one of the most beautiful ports in the Mediterranean. It is built on the ancient Kydonia, a town that existed until the end of the Second Byzantine period. The name "Hania" originally appeared during the Venetian occupation and became the most important administrative center of Western Crete. The Old Town was partially destroyed in 1645, during the Turkish occupation and was rebuilt again in 1840. The fortress, now a restaurant, dominates the entrance of the harbor and is the place where the flag of the Greek republic was hoisted in 1913. Today the port is as beautiful as ever! It is surrounded by quaint little shops, bountiful markets, and beautiful outdoor cafes offering healthy and delicious foods.

Baked Clams

24	large fresh clams
2	tablespoons extra virgin olive oil
½	cup finely chopped green onion
3	cloves garlic, finely chopped
2	tablespoons finely chopped parsley
½	teaspoon dried oregano
1	teaspoon hot sauce
½	cup breadcrumbs
2	lemons

Preheat oven to 400 degrees Fahrenheit.
Clean and shuck clams, and reserve the clam juice and the shells. Chop the clams and gather the remaining ingredients.

In a medium saucepan, heat the olive oil and sauté the chopped clams, onions and garlic over low heat. Remove the pan from the heat, and add the parsley, oregano, hot sauce, breadcrumbs and clam juice. Mix all the ingredients to moisten.

Using a tablespoon, fill the reserved shells with the clam mixture, place on a baking sheet and bake for 10 minutes. Squeeze fresh lemon juice on top before serving. Serves 6 appetizer portions.

To shuck clams: Place the clam in the palm of your hand, holding firm between the thumbs and index finger. Use a clam knife and line it up along the base of the shell, apply steady pressure until the knife slides in, and twist the knife to open the shell. Break off the top carefully not to lose the juice.

Shrimp with Garlic & Feta

1	lb jumbo shrimp (16 shrimp per lb)
½	teaspoon salt
¼	cup flour
¼	cup extra virgin olive oil
¼	cup finely chopped green onions
6	cloves garlic, crushed
2	tablespoons chopped ripe tomatoes
½	cup white wine
3	ounces feta cheese, crumbled
1	tablespoon finely chopped fresh parsley

Remove the shell from the shrimp, leaving the tail on, and devein; season with salt and lightly coat with flour.

In a large skillet, heat the olive oil over medium heat, sauté each side for 30 seconds, and transfer to a plate.

Add onions, tomatoes and garlic to the same skillet and sauté for 2-3 minutes. Return the shrimp to the skillet and add the wine, parsley and cheese. Continue to cook over low heat for another minute until the sauce thickens.

Transfer to a serving platter and squeeze fresh lemon juice on top of the shrimp. Serves 4

Chilled Shrimp & Crab Salad

½	lb shrimp (peeled, de-veined and cooked)
½	lb crabmeat, coarsely chopped
½	cup finely chopped celery leaves
½	cup finely chopped green onions
2	cloves garlic, crushed
¼	cup extra virgin olive oil
2	tablespoons freshly squeezed lemon juice
1	teaspoon hot sauce
¼	teaspoon salt
5	leaves romaine lettuce
1	lemon, sliced in wedges

Rinse the lettuce leaves under cold water and let them dry between paper towel layers. Layer a large serving platter with the lettuce leaves and place in the refrigerator to chill.

Chop the cooked shrimp into small pieces and place in a medium size bowl with the crabmeat, celery and onions.

In a small bowl combine the olive oil, crushed garlic, lemon juice, hot sauce, salt, and whisk to blend the ingredients. Pour over the seafood, tossing to coat the shrimp and crab with the dressing.

Place the seafood salad in the center of the serving platter, previously layered with the lettuce leaves, and garnish with lemon wedges. Serves 6

Baked Filet Of Halibut

2	lbs halibut filet (3/4 inch thick)
½	teaspoon salt
¼	teaspoon white pepper
½	cup onions, sliced thin
6	tablespoons olive oil
¼	cup chopped parsley
4	cloves garlic, finely chopped
2	tomatoes
	a few string of fresh rosemary

Preheat oven to 400 degrees Fahrenheit. Cut fish into six portions and place on a paper towel to dry.

Place the fish filets in a shallow baking-pan and season with olive oil, salt, pepper, parsley, garlic, onions and rosemary leaves.

Cut each tomato into three thick slices and place on top of each fish filet. Bake in a hot oven for 15-20 minutes. Serves 6

Filet of Sole with Almonds

2	lbs filet of Sole
½	teaspoon salt
2	tablespoons flour
6	tablespoons extra virgin olive oil
4	cloves garlic, sliced thin
½	cup slivered almonds
½	teaspoon sugar
1	lemon

Rinse the fish filets under cold water and let them dry between paper towel layers. Season the fish with salt and coat lightly with flour.

In a large skillet, heat the olive oil over medium heat and sauté the fish for one minute, turn to the other side and add the garlic slices continuing to sauté for another minute. Squeeze lemon juice on top of the fish transfer to serving platter.

Add the almonds and sugar to the same skillet, searing until the almonds are golden in color. Arrange the fish on the serving platter and garnish the top with the almonds. Serves 6

Mussels in Red Wine Sauce

½	cup olive oil
½	cup finely chopped onion
4	cloves chopped garlic
2	lbs ripe tomatoes, finely chopped
¼	cup finely chopped fresh basil
1	teaspoon salt
1	tablespoon hot sauce
½	cup chicken stock
2	lbs fresh mussels
½	cup red wine

Fresh mussels have a closed shell. Discard the mussels already opened and wash the remaining mussels in cold water, removing all the sand and seaweed from the shell.

In a large skillet, heat the olive oil and sauté the onions with the garlic for 1 to 2 minutes. Add the chopped tomatoes, basil, salt, stock, hot sauce and simmer for 5 minutes.

Add the mussels and wine, and simmer over medium heat until the shells open.

Spoon some of the sauce inside the shell and serve plain with fresh bread or over pasta. Serves 6

Seafood Chowder

1	2 lb whole Grouper, gutted and de-scaled
2	quarts water
1	teaspoon salt
6	small potatoes, peeled
3	small onions, peeled
1	celery stalk cut in half
3	strings of parsley
3	cloves garlic, peeled
2	ripe tomatoes, skin removed
3	carrots, peeled and cut in half
½	teaspoon white pepper
½	cup fresh squeezed lemon juice
½	cup extra virgin olive oil
½	lb shrimp
½	lb fresh mussels or clams

Place the fish in a large pot with the water and 1 tablespoon of salt over medium heat.

When it starts to boil, use a skimmer to remove the unwanted fat particles that surface to the top as the water boils. Cook the fish for 15 to 20 minutes or until tender. Using a large spatula, remove the fish from the pot to a serving platter carefully, to avoid breaking during the transfer.

Use a fine sieve to strain the stock into another pot and place the pot over low heat. Add the potatoes, onions, celery, parsley, tomatoes, carrots, garlic and pepper, and simmer for 30 minutes.

Add shrimp and mussels to the fish stock, and cook for 3-5 minutes until the mussels open their shells.

In a small bowl, combine olive oil and lemon juice, and beat lightly with a small whisk or fork.

Remove the skin and bones from the fish and pour half of the olive oil and lemon dressing on top

Serve a bowl of soup with one tablespoon of oil/lemon dressing, freshly chopped parsley and a piece of fish. Serves 8-10

Baked Salmon

2	lbs skinless salmon filet
3	tablespoons olive oil
4	cloves garlic, crushed
¼	cup finely chopped fresh dill
1	large red pepper, sliced in rings
½	teaspoon salt and a dash of pepper
1	lemon

Preheat oven to 400 degrees Fahrenheit.
Rinse salmon under cold water and cut into six equal portions.

Place in a shallow baking dish and season with salt, pepper, olive oil, garlic and dill, and arrange the red pepper ring on top.

Bake for 15 minutes in the preheated oven. Remove from oven, transfer to a large platter and squeeze fresh lemon juice on top. Serves 6

Belgium Endives Stuffed with Salmon

1	lb fresh salmon filet, skin removed
½	cup white wine
¼	teaspoon salt
½	lb of Belgium endives
4	tablespoons olive oil
1	tablespoon lemon juice and lemon slices
¼	cup chopped walnuts
1	tablespoon freshly chopped dill
1	teaspoon of hot sauce
1	tablespoon of small capers

Wash the endive leaves, tear apart gently and place on a large platter. Salt the salmon filet and steam in a medium saucepan with the wine for 5-8 minutes (cooking time depends on the thickness of the filet).

Place the steamed salmon in a bowl and break into small pieces with a fork. Add the olive oil, lemon juice, walnuts, hot sauce, capers and half of the dill. Mix well to blend all the ingredients.

Using a tablespoon, fill the Belgium endive leaves with the salmon mixture and garnish with the remaining chopped dill and the lemon slices. Chill for 2 hours before serving. Serves 4-6

Salmon Glazed with Honey & Almonds

2	lbs skinless salmon filet
¼	cup extra virgin olive oil
¼	cup finely chopped onion
½	teaspoon salt
¼	teaspoon freshly ground pepper
1	cup white wine
2	tablespoons finely chopped fresh thyme
1	tablespoon of honey
1	teaspoon prepared mustard
½	cup sliced almonds
1	lemon cut in wedges

For the greens:

½	lb of mixed greens, pre-washed and chilled
1	ounce fresh watercress, chopped coarsely
1	sour apple, cored and sliced very thin
2	tablespoons extra virgin olive oil
1	tablespoon balsamic vinegar
1	clove garlic, crushed
	salt and pepper to taste

In a large bowl combine the mixed greens, watercress, sliced apple, olive oil, vinegar, crushed garlic, salt and pepper, and toss. Transfer to large serving platter and chill.

In a small bowl combine the wine, thyme, honey, mustard, and whisk to blend the ingredients. Set *aside. Cut the salmon in 6 equal portions and season with salt and pepper.*

In a large non-stick skillet, heat the olive oil over low heat and sear the salmon on both sides for 1 minute, add the onions, and sauté another minute.

Add the wine mixture to the salmon, cover, and simmer for 3 minutes. Add the almonds and cook uncovered 2 minutes to glaze the almonds.

Arrange the glazed salmon on top of the greens and sliced sour apple salad. Garnish with the almonds and lemon wedges. Serves 6

Sea bass & Scallops in White Wine Sauce

1	lb sea Bass filet
½	lb sea scallops
½	teaspoon salt
¼	teaspoon cayenne pepper
¼	cup flour
4	tablespoons olive oil
¼	cup finely chopped fresh chives
2	cloves garlic, crushed
½	ounce fresh thyme leaves
½	cup white wine
½	cup chicken stock

Cut the sea Bass in four equal portions. Season the seafood pieces with salt and lightly flour.

Heat the olive oil and sauté the scallops and fish filets for 1-2 minute on each side. Add the chives, garlic, thyme, cayenne pepper, wine and stock. Cover and simmer for 3 minutes. Serve with cooked angel hair pasta. Serves 4

Tip: The wine can be substituted for more stock.

Baked Trout

4	12-ounce fresh whole trout, de-scaled and gutted
	salt and pepper to taste
¼	cup extra virgin olive oil
2	tablespoons flat leaf parsley
¼	cup fresh lemon juice

Preheat oven to 400 degrees Fahrenheit.
Season the trout with salt and pepper, and coat with one tablespoon of the olive oil. Take a large piece of foil, line the inside of the foil with wax paper and place the trout on top of the wax paper. Enclose the foil and place it in a shallow baking pan. Bake for 20 minutes.

To test if the fish is cooked, insert a knife in the center of the fattest part of the fish. The flesh close to the bone should be white; if it's still pink, it needs a little more time to cook. The flesh should come off the bone easily.

In a small bowl combine the remaining olive oil, parsley and lemon juice and whisk lightly with a fork to blend the ingredients.

Place the cooked fish on a platter, de-bone gently, and pour the olive oil and lemon mixture on top. Serve with Greek Salad. Serves 4

CHAPTER 12

The Sweets Shop

Remember, you can visit the bakery or sweets shop occasionally. You may prepare your choice of dessert from this chapter on a special occasion and limit your consumption to <u>one portion</u>.

Baklava

1	lb finely chopped walnuts
1	tsp ground cinnamon
2	tablespoons sugar
1	lb fillo pastry dough
6	ounces melted butter

Syrup:

½	cup honey
1	cup sugar
3	cups water
1	cinnamon stick
5	cloves
1	slice orange
1	ounce brandy

Defrost the phyllo pastry according to the package directions, at least two hours prior to preparing the dessert, and preheat the oven to 325 degrees Fahrenheit.

In a small bowl combine the walnuts, cinnamon sugar, and melt the butter in the microwave for 20 seconds or in a small saucepan over low heat.

Using a pastry brush, grease the bottom and sides of a 13X11X2 inch pan with melted butter. Unfold the phyllo pastry and layer the bottom of the pan, one leaf at a time, brushing each leaf with melted butter until one fourth of the phyllo pastry has been used.

Sprinkle 1/3 the walnut mixture on the top of the layered pastry evenly and continue the process layering two to three pastry leaves between the walnut layers. Use 6-8 leaves of pastry for the top layer and use the pastry brush to tuck the pastry ends toward the inside of the pan.

Using a sharp knife, cut the phyllo layers starting from the top all the way through to the bottom of the pan diagonally, approximately 1½ inches in width, creating 14 diamond shape pieces (hold the pastry down with the one hand while you cut with the other hand). Bake in a preheated oven for 1-½ hours or until color is golden. <u>Do not cover during cooking or after</u>.

While the dessert is baking, prepare the honey syrup by combining all the ingredients in a small saucepan. Simmer for 20 minutes and set aside to cool.

Remove the baklava from the oven and drizzel <u>cooled</u> syrup over the top slowly and evenly, and let it stand in room temperature 1 hour before serving. Serves 14

Butter Cookies

2	cups sweet butter
1	cup sugar
2	eggs
1	teaspoon vanilla
2	teaspoons baking powder
5	cups sifted cake flour
½	cup blanched almonds, chopped

Topping: ½   cup powdered sugar

Preheat oven to 350 degrees Fahrenheit. Beat butter and sugar with an electric mixer for 3 minutes until light and fluffy. Add eggs, vanilla and continue beating 2 minutes.

Sift together the flour and baking powder, and add half of the flour to the butter mixture while beating on the low speed. Add remaining flour, while mixing by hand to form a soft dough, and blend in the almonds.

Pinch off a small portion of the dough and shape into a small cookie in the shape of a half moon or a three pointed star.

Place the cookies in a baking sheet and bake for 20-25 minutes until golden. Remove from oven and sift powdered sugar over the cookies while they are still hot. Makes 4-5 dozen depending on the size. Serving portion is 2 cookies.

Honey Macaroons

½	cup sugar
1	cup butter
3	eggs
½	cup orange juice
1	tablespoon orange rind
1	teaspoon baking soda
½	teaspoon ground cinnamon
¼	teaspoon ground cloves
4	cups all-purpose flour
½	cup finely chopped walnuts

Graze: *Prepare the syrup as described in the recipe for the Baklava.*

Preheat oven to 375 degrees Fahrenheit. Cream together butter, eggs and sugar for 3 minutes with an electric mixer. Add the orange rind, juice, baking soda, and continue beating for 1 minute.

Sift together the flour, cinnamon, nuts and ground cloves. Add the flour mixture to the eggs, and using your hands, mix until you form a soft dough. You may need additional flour, but be careful not to add too much as the cookie dough should be soft.

Pinch off a tablespoon of dough and form it into long oblong shape macaroon, placing each macaroon on a baking sheet approximately two inches apart.

Use a fork, press the top of the macaroons to flatten and pierce through the dough to make little holes (this process will permit the honey syrup to penetrate the macaroon during glazing). Bake for 30 minutes or until golden.

Cool on a wire rack and prepare the honey syrup and walnut mixture. Makes 4-dozen depending on the size. Serve 2 macaroons per person.

Walnut Mix:

½ lb walnuts, finely chopped
1 teaspoon ground cinnamon
1 tablespoon granulated sugar

Dip 3 or 4 cooled macaroons in syrup while it's simmering for 30 seconds.

Use a slotted spatula to remove the macaroons from the hot syrup, gently transferring them to a serving platter.

Sprinkle a ½ teaspoon of the walnut mixture on top of each macaroon immediately after glazing.

Tip: If the syrup becomes thick during simmer, lower the temperature and add one ounce water.

Apples Baked in Phyllo Pastry

This dessert is my absolute favorite! I developed this recipe several years ago for my restaurant. I wanted a dessert that was not very sweet and could be served with frozen yogurt or vanilla ice cream. Serve hot out of the oven with a scoop of low-fat vanilla yogurt.

For the filling:

6	large apples, cored, peeled and sliced
¼	cup sugar
1	tablespoon cornstarch
1	teaspoon ground cinnamon
1	tablespoon melted butter

For the pastry:

½	lb phyllo pastry
¼	cup butter, melted
1	tablespoon of cinnamon sugar mixture

Defrost the phyllo pastry and preheat oven to 375 degrees Fahrenheit.

Mix together the sugar, cornstarch and cinnamon. Place sliced apples in a large bowl, add the melted butter and coat the apples evenly using a large spoon. Add the dry ingredients and toss.

Use a pastry brush to grease a 10X3 inch deep baking pan with melted butter.

Layer the bottom of the baking pan with eight layers of the pastry, coating each pastry layer lightly with melted butter. Allow three pastry sheets to overlap the sides of the pan.

Place the apple filling in the pan and fold over the overlapping pastry. Layer the remaining pastry on top, and sprinkle with cinnamon and sugar. Bake for 1 hour. Serves 8

Rice Pudding

1	cup water
½	cup rice
4	cups milk, warmed
1	teaspoon vanilla
1	teaspoon cornstarch
1	cup sugar
3	eggs
	a pinch of ground cinnamon

In a medium sauce pan, combine water and rice. Cook over low heat for 20 minutes. Add the warm milk, stir, and continue simmering for 2 hours, stirring occasionally to prevent sticking.

Beat the eggs, sugar, vanilla and cornstarch with an electric mixer until it becomes fluffy. Add the egg mixture to the hot milk and stir gently until the pudding thickens. Remove from heat and use a ladle to fill 6 small bowls with the pudding. Sprinkle with cinnamon before serving.

Spanish Custard

2	cups hot milk
3	large eggs
½	cup sugar
1	teaspoon vanilla extract

For the caramel:

1	teaspoon water
6	tablespoons sugar

Place the six tablespoons of sugar and teaspoon of water in a small saucepan. Heat over low heat, stirring until the sugar turns into golden syrup, and immediately pour into four small ramekin cups. Set aside and preheat oven to 325 degrees Fahrenheit.

In a heavy saucepan, heat the milk to scalding, but not boiling. In a large mixing bowl beat eggs, sugar, and vanilla with an electric mixer; slowly add hot milk, and whisk gently until the milk is blended.

Using a ladle, fill the caramel coated ramekin cups with the hot milk mixture and place the cups in a shallow baking pan with a half inch deep in water bath. Bake until custard is firm and the surface turns golden, approximately 40 minutes. Chill before serving. Serves 4

Semolina Custard with Raspberries

6	cups milk
2	tablespoons butter
1	cup semolina
1	cup granulated sugar
6	eggs
1	teaspoon vanilla

Topping:

1	tablespoon powdered sugar
2	cups fresh raspberries

Preheat oven to 350 degrees Fahrenheit. Brush a 10X10X3-inch baking pan with melted butter.

Combine the milk, butter and semolina in a large saucepot. Place the pot over medium-low heat and stir continually with a whisk to prevent clumping and sticking, until the mixture is thick. Remove from heat.

Beat the eggs, vanilla and granulated sugar until thick. Add to the hot milk, stirring quickly with a whisk to blend the eggs evenly. Remove the custard from the heat and pour into the greased baking pan. Bake in a preheated oven for 30-40 minutes.

Cool, dust lightly with powdered sugar and arrange the fresh berries on top. Serves 8

Walnut Cake

4	eggs
¾	cup sugar
¾	cup butter, soften
1	teaspoon vanilla
1	cup flour
2	teaspoons baking powder
1	teaspoon ground cinnamon
½	teaspoon ground cloves
1	cup finely chopped walnuts
1	ounce brandy

Preheat oven to 350 degrees Fahrenheit.
Mix together the flour, baking powder, cinnamon and cloves. Set aside, and separate egg white and egg yolks in two separate bowls.

In a mixing bowl beat the egg white to soft peaks.

In separate bowl combine sugar, butter, vanilla, and egg yolks. Beat with an electric mixer on high speed for 2 minutes, reduce to low speed, and fold in the eggs whites alternately with the dry ingredients and brandy blending.

Pour in 10X10X2-inch lightly greased baking pan. Bake in the preheated oven for 35-40 minutes (insert a toothpick in the center of the cake, if it come out clean the cake is completely cooked). Remove from the oven and cool on a wire rack. Serves 8

Yogurt Cake

½   cup butter, soften
12 ounces plain yogurt
1   cup sugar
1   teaspoon vanilla
5   eggs
2   cups cake flour
2   teaspoons baking powder

Toppings:

1   tablespoon powdered sugar
2   cups fresh strawberries

Preheat oven to 350 degrees Fahrenheit.
Sift flour and baking powder into a small bowl. In a large mixing bowl, beat the butter, sugar, eggs and vanilla with an electric mixer for 3 minutes. Add yogurt alternately with the flour mixture and continue mixing on low speed until well blended.

Brush a 10X3 inch round cake pan lightly with melted butter and pour in the yogurt mixture. Bake in the preheated oven for 45 minutes.

Before serving, garnish with powdered sugar and fresh strawberries. Serves 8

Bread Pudding

2	cups milk, scalded
6	ounces French bread sliced thin
1	tablespoon unsalted butter, melted
½	cup sugar
4	eggs
½	teaspoon pure vanilla
½	cup sliced fresh strawberries, raspberries or apricots

Preheat oven to 350 degrees Fahrenheit.
Melt the butter and slice the bread. Use a pastry brush to coat the bread slices lightly with melted butter.

In a medium-size bowl combine the sugar, eggs, vanilla, and beat lightly with an electric mixer. Add the hot milk to the eggs, blending gently.

Line the bread slices in a deep baking dish (8X8X3 inches deep) and pour the egg mixture over the bread. Push the bread down with a spoon to soak in the bread with the milk mixture, cover, and bake for 25 minutes. Add the fruit on top of the bread pudding and bake 10 minutes longer. Serve hot or cold. Serves 6

Crepes with Yogurt & Berries

1½   cup all-purpose flour
2   eggs
1   teaspoon vanilla extract
1   tablespoon sugar
1   cup milk
2   tablespoons melted butter for grilling

For the filling:

2   cups sliced berries
1   shot of cognac
1   teaspoon granulated sugar
1   cup low-fat yogurt
1   tablespoon powdered sugar for topping

Sift the flour into a large mixing bowl. Add the eggs, sugar, milk, vanilla, and beat with an electric mixer or whisk until the batter is thick and free of lumps.
Using a non-stick crepe pan or a small frying pan, place a ½ teaspoon of butter in the frying pan over medium heat. As soon as the butter melts, add 2 tablespoons of crepe batter, tilting the pan so that it spreads across the bottom surface to make a round crepe; hold for 15 seconds until it turns golden brown, and turn over to brown the other side.

Place the finished crepes between two pieces of wax paper until they are ready to be served.

In a small bowl, combine the granulated sugar, cognac and sliced berries. Place two tablespoons of yogurt in the center of each crepe topped with two tablespoons of sliced berries and fold. Sprinkle the top with powdered sugar before serving. Serves 6

Donut Puffs with Honey & Nuts

2	cups lukewarm water
2	cups all-purpose flour
1	teaspoon sugar
1	teaspoon active dry yeast
2	cups corn oil for frying

Topping:

¼	cup warm honey
1	teaspoon ground cinnamon
¼	cup finely chopped pecans

In a small bowl, combine the water, flour, sugar, and yeast, and blend well. Cover with a towel and let it rise for 30 minutes. In a medium non-stick saucepan, heat the corn oil. Using a tablespoon, drop a spoonful of dough into the hot oil; the dough will fall to the bottom of the pan and puff back up to the surface, as it cooks. Turn with a slotted spoon and let it fry until golden. Pour 5-6 spoonfuls of soft dough in the oil at one time. Transfer the cooked puffs on a plate lined with paper towel. Drizzle warm honey over puffs, and sprinkle with cinnamon and nuts. Makes 24. Serves 4

Easter Sweet Bread

2	envelopes fast acting dry yeast
½	cup warm water
2	cups milk, lukewarm
1	cup sweet butter, softened
2	cups granulated sugar
6	eggs
1	teaspoon vanilla
12	cups sifted all-purpose flour

Topping:

2	egg yolks
¼	cup water
¼	teaspoon vanilla
3	hardboiled eggs, dyed red
3	tablespoons slivered almonds

Preheat oven to 350 degrees Fahrenheit.
Soften the yeast in the warm water and let the eggs stay in room temperature 30 minutes prior to preparation. Beat the butter, sugar and vanilla for 3 minutes on high speed, add eggs, and continue beating until fluffy. Add softened yeast, milk, and 4 cups of the flour. Continue beating with the electric mixer 1-2 minutes.

Place the remaining flour in a large bowl, add the egg mixture, and knead until you have soft and pliable dough. You may add more or less flour if necessary. Cover with a damp cloth and let rise the dough rise until double; punch down again to shape into three loaves. Place each loaf on baking sheet lined with wax paper and cover with a towel until doubled in bulk, about two hours. Decorate the loaves with a red egg and bake for 20 minutes. In a small bowl beat the egg yolks, vanilla and water. Bring the loaves out of the oven to brush the tops with the egg mixture, sprinkle with almonds and return to the oven for 15 minutes.

Banana Zucchini Bread

1 ½	cup all-purpose flour
1	teaspoon baking powder
½	teaspoon ground cinnamon
¼	cup finely chopped nuts
½	cup sugar
2	eggs
¼	cup Canola oil
½	cup mashed bananas
½	cup finely shredded zucchini

Preheat oven to 350 degrees Fahrenheit. In a small bowl sift the flour, baking powder and cinnamon and add the nuts. In a separate bowl, beat the sugar and oil for 2 minutes with an electric mixer and add the eggs, one at a time; beat until smooth.

Fold in the flour alternately with the zucchini and bananas until moisten. Pour the batter into a lightly greased loaf pan (8X4X2-inch). Bake for 45 minutes. Serves 8.

New Year's Day Cake

1	cup butter
1	cup sugar
1	teaspoon pure vanilla
5	eggs, separated
¼	cup orange juice
1	teaspoon fresh orange rind
2	cups cake flour
2	teaspoons baking powder
¼	cup slivered almonds
¼	cup powdered sugar

Preheat oven to 350 degrees Fahrenheit.
Sift together the flour and baking powder, and separate the egg yolks from egg whites in two different bowls. Beat the egg whites to soft peaks.

Cream together the butter, sugar, orange rind, egg yolks and vanilla with an electric mixer until the texture becomes thick. Add the flour, alternately with the orange juice, beating on low speed until all the ingredients have been well blended. Using a spatula, fold the egg whites into the batter gently.

Pour the cake batter in a 9X3-inch cake pan and sprinkle sliced almonds on the top. Bake for 50 minutes. The center of the cake should be slightly cracked or firm before removing from oven. Sift powdered sugar on top and serve. Serves 8

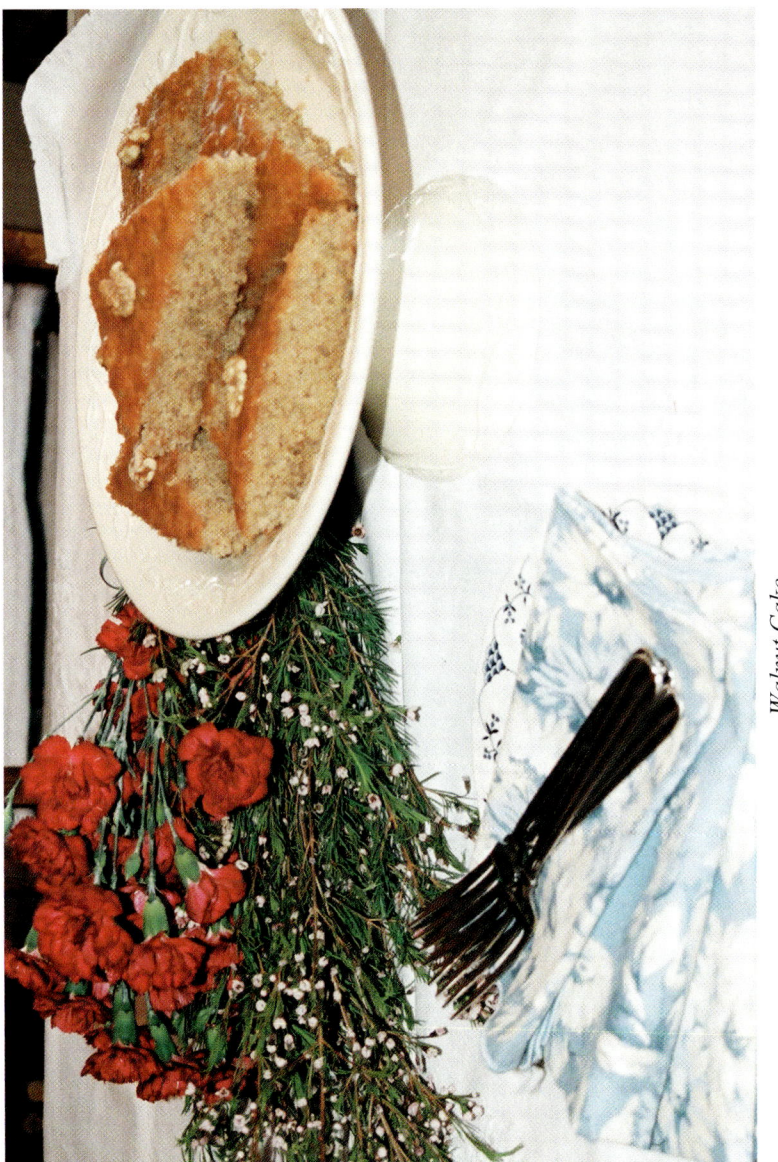

Walnut Cake

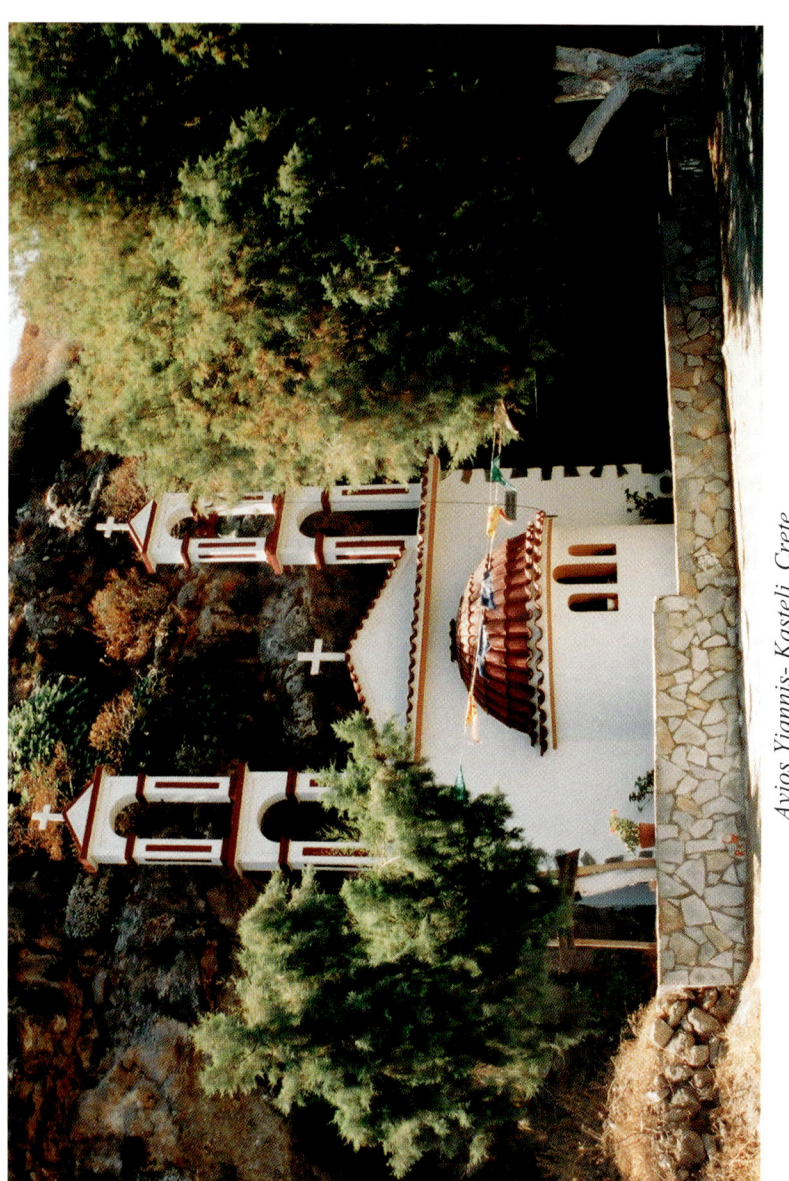

Ayios Yiannis- Kasteli, Crete

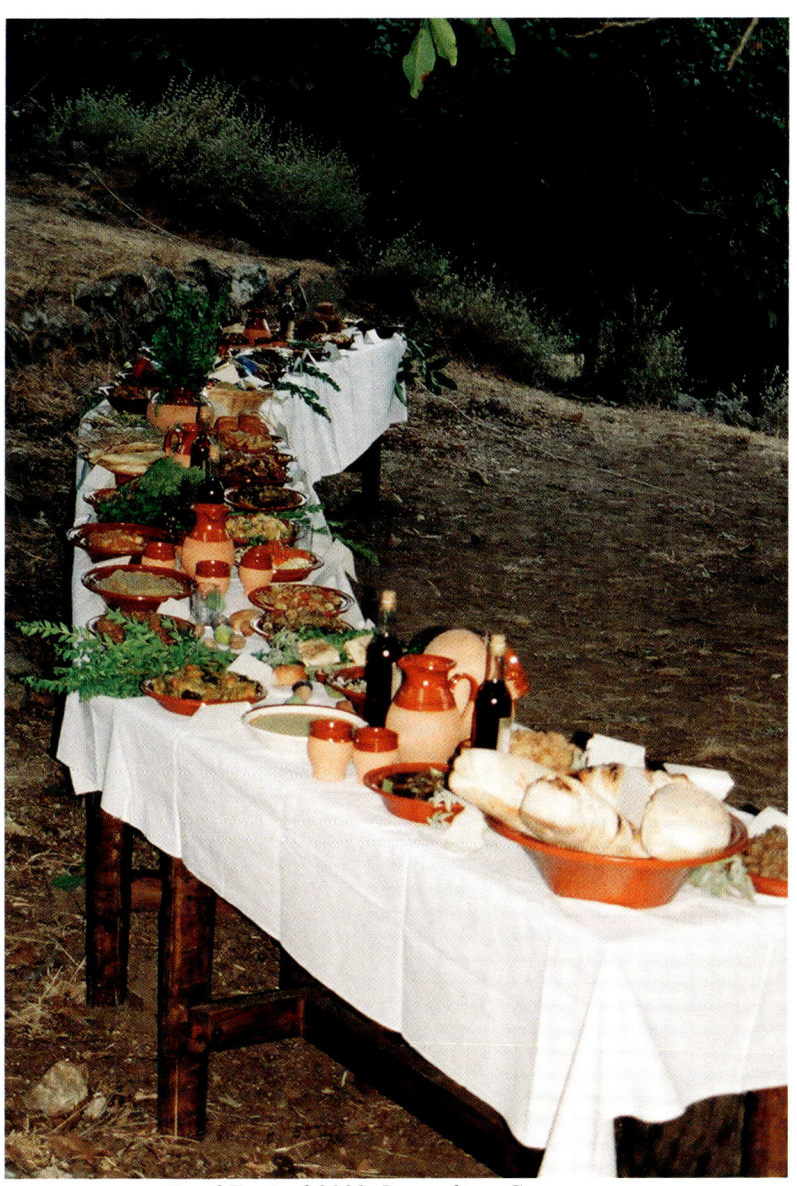

Food Festival 2000, Loussakies, Crete

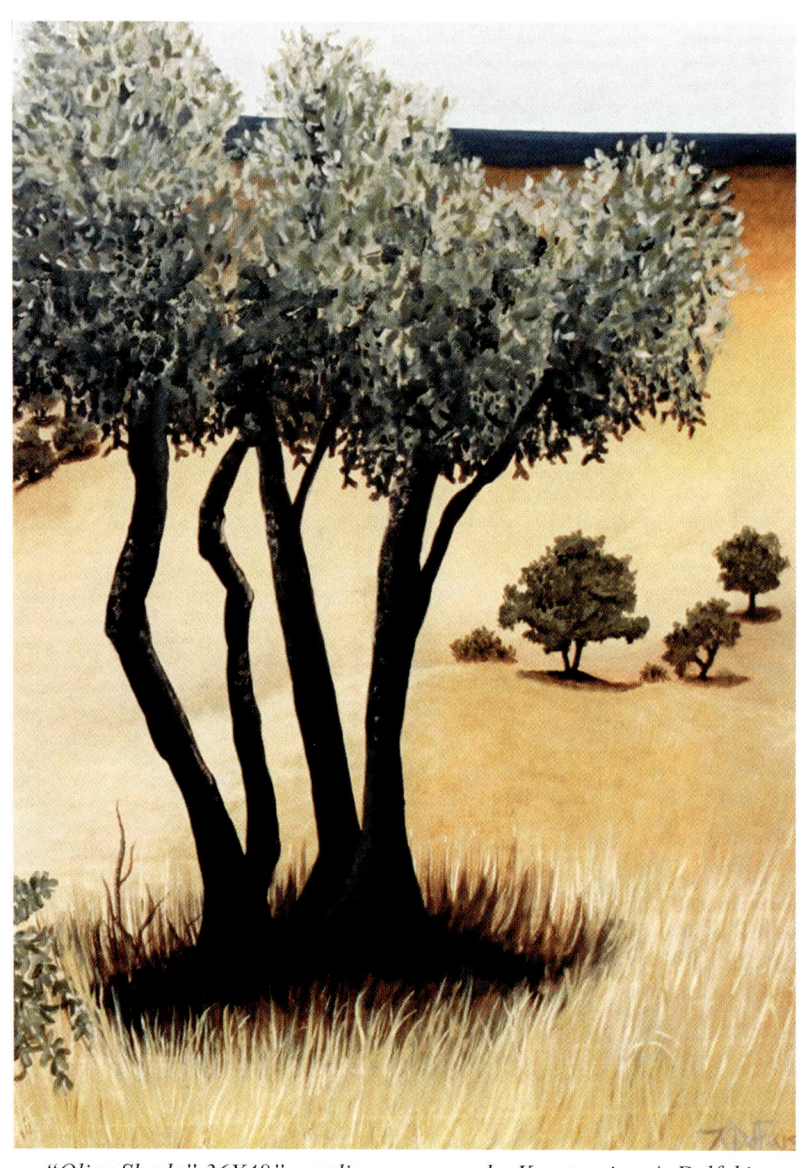

"Olive Shade" 36X48" acrylic on canvas, by Konstantina A. Delfakis

Herbal Remedies Alcohol & Caffeine Consumption

CHAPTER 13

HERBAL REMEDIES

Herbs have been admired for their beauty and fragrance, consumed for their flavor and curative properties, used in cosmetics and dyes, and as aphrodisiacs for thousands of years.
Theophrastus, a Greek herbalist and a student of Aristotle and Plato, was considered the father of botany (371-287 BC). He wrote the first book on plants titled "History of Plants", which contained 450 plants in systematic categories, including the plant's origin. He was the first herbalist to have his own garden and later, after Alexander the Great conquered Persia, gardens flourished throughout Greece and Rome. Most European medicine began from the Romans who received their training and knowledge for herbs from two Greek doctors: Galen, a physician to Marcus Aurelius, and Dioscorides, a physician who traveled with the Roman legions and who wrote the first true herbal "De Materia Medica," a manuscript containing 500 Mediterranean area medicinal plants and their functions. Galen, Dioscorides and Theophrastus were authorities of European herbalism and herbal medicine, during the first and second century A.D.

Since the early 1990's we have seen a four-fold increase in the usage of herb remedies as

Americans try to treat their own health problems; colds, flu, pain, allergies, memory loss depression, premenstrual syndrome, menopause and many other ailments. We spend twice the amount of money on herbs as we do on vitamins, exceeding five billion dollars annually. Every year more of us are searching for alternative medicines because we are dissatisfied with the current medical care that they are receiving. Other reasons for the increased herb usage include the continued increased cost of health care, the over-dependence that doctors and other clinicians place on medical technology, and the impersonal way that most physicians treat their patients. In addition, very few physicians know about herbs and fail to acknowledge the literature on some of their benefits, as another option to medical treatment.

Most people see herb remedies as a safe option of treatment and prevention. In addition, herbal remedies can be purchased without a prescription, making them more accessible than traditional medicines. Each year however, many people experience the bad side of herbs with mild to severe consequences, including death. Most people are unaware of the dangerous side effects of herbal remedies and unintentionally abuse their use, especially when they take them with other medications. Many herbs used for medical purposes in many countries around the world are unavailable in the United States. The herbs imported to the U.S however, have a tremendous impact on our health. In this chapter, I will outline the most popular herbs used in the U.S today, their benefits and their side effects.

POPULAR HERBAL REMEDIES

Chamomile is one the most popular and safest herb in the world. The daisy-like blossoms with their apple fragrance have been used to relieve menstrual symptoms, to stimulate appetite and promote digestion, and as a sleeping aid. Chamomile is consumed mostly as tea, but it is also considered an important ingredient in beauty products such as skin creams, shampoos, hand lotions and hair highlighter. The benefits of chamomile consumption include improved digestion, relaxation, sleep and to sooths the skin.
Side effects: An allergic reaction to chamomile is possible and it may aggravate people with hay fever by causing an itching sensation in the mouth and throat. People who suffer with allergies or hay fever should avoid drinking chamomile tea.

Echinacea was used by Native Americans to cure snakebites and bites from poisonous insects, tumors, syphilis, gangrene, hemorrhoids and eczema. They also used the juice of the plant to cure burns. Early American Settlers used echinacea to fight against the flu and virus. Many herbalists still consider echinacea a blood purifier and an effective antibiotic; its benefits may include strengthening the immune system to fight against colds, flu and respiratory infections.
Side effects: Most clinicians agree that echinacea should not be taken for more than six weeks at a time and people with autoimmune disorders should avoid taking it.

Feverfew *was used by Europeans to reduce headache, fever and relief from arthritis, and during the ancient times, it was used to relieve menstrual symptoms. In the seventeenth century it was used to treat "female hysteria" known today as PMS (Post Menstrual Syndrome), infant colic, depression, kidney stones, constipation and insect bites. Today, it is most commonly used to treat migraine headaches. Be careful when taking feverfew, eating the leaves may result in swelling of the mouth, lips and tongue, and ulcerations in the mouth. In addition, be very cautious when combining with other medications.*

Ginseng *is commonly available as Korean ginseng or Siberian ginseng. Korean ginseng is processed from the plant's root, and the Siberian ginseng is processed from the plant's root and leaves. Ginseng has been used by the Chinese to increase strength, stamina and promote longevity. The Korean ginseng has been promoted as an aphrodisiac, but this claim has not been proven. Benefits from taking ginseng may include increased energy levels, relieve symptoms of mild depression, increase endurance, strengthen the immune response and improve mental alertness.*
Side effects: May cause increase in blood pressure, restlessness, nervousness, headaches, diarrhea skin problems, palpitations and tremor. In some women it can cause breast pain or uterine bleeding. Women with breast cancer should avoid taking this herb. In addition, ginseng may cause a hypoglycemic effect in diabetic patients on insulin, and it can be dangerous for people who have

hypertension, headaches, heart arrhythmias or thyroid disorders.

Ginkgo Biloba is commonly used in China and Europe to cure problems with blood circulation and memory loss. Possible benefits include improving blood flow to the brain, memory and peripheral. Ginkgo biloba may improve erectile function in men who suffer from impotence and decrease pain in people with vascular disease.
Ginkgo may cause intestinal problems in some people and other serious complications, such as bleeding around the brain or under the skull. In addition, people who are taking blood-thinning medications or have bleeding disorders should avoid taking this herb. Do not take with aspirin, ibuprofen, arthritis drugs or high dozes of vitamin E.

Goldenseal Cherokee Indians used the juice of the herb to stain their faces and cloths to prevent from being recognized as red men. Goldenseal is a natural antibiotic with antiseptic and anti-fungal properties. This herb has been used by Native Americans to cure mouth sores, eye irritations, and reduce swelling from infections and allergies. Currently, many people use goldenseal to reduce fever and headache pain, but there is no scientific evidence to support these benefits. Goldenseal may help in treating canker sores and other ulcers of the mouth. Side effects may include mouth irritations, nausea and vomiting, hypertension, convulsions and respiratory failure. Pregnant and lactating mothers should avoid taking this herb; its benefits have not been proven and the side effects are too dangerous to ignore.

Milk Thistle has been very popular in Germany for the treatment of liver disease; it reacts as an antioxidant by increasing protein synthesis in the liver, thus promoting normal liver function. Possible benefits include help in treating chronic liver disease.
Some individuals may experience diarrhea after a few days of treatment and it be harmful to people with hepatitis or cirrhosis of the liver.

Saw Palmetto is widely used in Europe for the treatment of benign prostate tumors. Benefits include treating urinary tract symptoms such as urinary frequency, hesitation, nighttime urination and discomfort when urinating.
Saw palmetto may be very harmful to men taking hormonal drugs for prostate disease.

Valerian Root is known to induce calmness in the brain center, and it has been used to treat insomnia and anxiety. Its benefits include improved sleep and reduction of anxiety.
However, prolonged intake of valerian root can cause coordination problems, a decrease in body temperature, depression, increased heart rate and headaches. This herb should not be taken with medications, especially sedatives or tranquilizers.

Kava-Kava was first brought to the west by captain Cook from one of his voyages to the South Pacific. Studies in Germany have shown that this herb is helpful in treating anxiety disorders in pre-

and post-menopausal women. The benefits of kava-kava include improved muscle relaxation, better control of pain and relief from anxiety symptoms.
Side effects may include scaly dry skin or rash, and gastro intestinal discomfort. Excessive use of this herb can result in dizziness, eye irritations, and discoloration of the hair and nails. Additionally, kava-kava should not be consumed by people with chronic depression, or taken with medications and supplements.

St John's-wort *has been popular in Europe for centuries. It is believed to increase resistance to colds and flu, induce weight loss, and help fight against depression and anxiety symptoms. In Germany, St John's-wort is prescribed as often as Prozac. Benefits may include improved sleep and relief from depression.*
Side effects include dizziness and dry mouth, anxiety and skin sensitivity to light. If St. John's-wort is combined with anti-depressants and decongestant drugs, it may cause serious life threatening complications.

DANGEROUS HERBS

Blue Cohosh has a toxic effect on the heart muscle and intestines, and may cause intestinal spasms, increase in blood pressure and heart failure. Blue Cohosh should never be used for medical self-treatment.

Comfrey contains substances that depress the central nervous system. Both the leaves and the root are carcinogenic. Taken orally it can cause toxicity to the liver and cancer.

Deadly Nightshade is an extremely poisonous! Poisoning manifests within 15 minutes of ingestion by dry mouth, burning of the throat, dilated pupils, intense thirst, double vision, rapid pulse, nausea and hallucinations.

Ephedra is a dangerous herb and should not be consumed by anyone, especially people with diabetes, heart disease, high blood pressure and thyroid disease.

Foxglove. People have died from ingestion of foxglove. The symptoms of foxglove poisoning include nausea, diarrhea, migraine headache, stomach pain, irregular heartbeat, tremors, convulsions and death.

Juniper Even small repeated doses can cause convulsions and kidney damage.

Jimsonweed *may cause hallucinations and death. Symptoms may also include dimness of vision, delirium, giddiness and mania.*

Life Root *was used in the past during childbirth for pain. Causes liver toxicity and uterine bleeding in women.*

Lobelia *is a very dangerous herb that has been used to aid in weight loss. Symptoms include severe nausea, thus the reason for the weight loss. Lobelia may be fatal.*

Mistletoe. *Do not kiss it! Consumption of the berries or leaves of the plant can cause irregular heartbeat and death.*

Sassafras. *Even a very small amount of the herb's volatile oils can cause breakdown of the heart, liver and kidneys. It has also been found to increase the risk of cancer.*

Tropical Periwinkle *is a source of chemotherapy drugs. It is extremely powerful and even a small dose can be very harmful.*

Pokeroot *is harmful. Claims of its curative properties for cancer and rheumatism have not been substantiated.*

Many people are looking into curing themselves of disease by self-medicating with herbs, hoping to improve their health or cure their illness and stop the aging process. Most of these claims are fraudulent. <u>Be careful</u>, educate yourself about the *herbs you plan to consume and ask a professional for advice. Look out for phrases such as "encourages rejuvenation", "strengthens the body", "detoxifies the body", "purifies the blood" and many others. These companies spend a lot of money on researching what people want to hear.*

Some herbs can be helpful in relieving disease symptoms, but keep in mind that herbs are like medications and just because they are natural, does not mean they are safe. There are thousands of plants on the earth and many of them are naturally poisonous. Many of our medications are made from natural plants, but we do not take them without a doctor's prescription. Therefore, why take herbs without a prescription? Furthermore, combining herbs with vitamins, medications and alcohol can be very dangerous! People who take herbal remedies should consider taking them in the smallest dose and only one at a time. Taking one herb at a time in the minimum dose is a good way to identify the herb that might have an adverse effect.

What You Should Consider Before Taking Herb Remedies

- *Choose herb products produced by reputable companies.*

- *Buy pure products, not the cheapest brand. Cultivation and production of herbs in a pure form is very expensive.*

- *Before taking herbal remedies, talk it over with a professional who is knowledgeable on the subject, especially if herbs are to be taken with other medications.*

- *Do not combine herbs with vitamins or medications.*

- *Take herb medications one at a time and for a short period of time, not long-term.*

- *Do not give herbal medications to children.*

- *Pregnant women and nursing mothers should not take herbal remedies, because they may penetrate the placenta and milk supply.*

CHAPTER 14

THE FACTS ABOUT ALCOHOL

Fourteen million Americans are either dependent on alcohol or they abuse its use daily. Most families are affected by at least one member having an alcohol related problem. Alcohol consumption causes 40% of all fatal traffic accidents and is the number one cause of death among teenagers. In the U.S., 33% of all hospital admissions and 20% of all healthcare costs are attributed to the use of alcohol. Research studies show that heavy drinking (more than two drinks per day) of alcoholic beverages increases the risk of many types of cancers, especially if the person is smoking. Excessive alcohol consumption has been linked to:

- *Cancer of the colon, liver, breast, tracheal and oral cavity*
- *Osteoporosis in post-menopausal women*
- *High blood pressure*
- *Poor coordination, insomnia, depression and decreased cognitive function in the elderly*
- *Female infertility*
- *Nutrient deficiencies*
- *Traffic and other accidents*
- *Domestic violence*

The risk of breast cancer in women increases at two drinks per day. Fortunately, only a few women in the U.S. exceed one drink per day and only about two percent of the breast cancer cases are attributed to alcohol consumption. On the other hand, studies in Europe, where women consume more alcohol than American women, show a five-fold increase in breast cancer cases.

Alcohol abuse problems are more common among men than they are among women. However, the risk of health problems and intoxication is greater among women for several reasons:

1. *Women tend to have more fat and less body water and since alcohol is water soluble, the concentration of alcohol in their blood is higher.*

2. *As women age; they accumulate additional body fat and lose more water, therefore, more easily intoxicated from alcohol.*

3. *Body weight is also important in tolerating alcohol and since women generally weigh less, their tolerance is lower than that of men.*

4. *The enzyme alcohol dehydrogenase (found in the stomach) plays an important role in metabolizing alcohol. Women tend to have less of this enzyme, and are therefore less able to metabolize alcohol.*

Of all the alcohol consumed as a beverage in the United States, 13% is consumed as spirits, 57% is consumed as beer and 13% is consumed as wine. Because of the high risks of cancer, heart disease and the many deaths attributed to alcohol abuse, it is important to take drinking alcoholic beverages seriously. Even moderate drinking can be harmful for some people, and we do not know enough to give advice those who currently do not drink, to start moderate drinking as a health benefit.

Many things can cause the body to go into what is called "Oxidative Stress" caused when the body produces small molecules, "free radicals," that can cause damage to the arteries, cancer and many other health problems. We know for example, that smoking causes damage to the cells by oxidative stress. Excessive alcohol consumption causes oxidative stress, but unlike smoking, it can also act as an antioxidant, if consumed in moderation. Recent studies show that moderate drinking of alcohol appears to have the antioxidant effect on the body. However, the findings vary among different population groups and type of alcohol that is consumed. Most researchers agree that moderate alcohol consumption reduces the risk of stroke and heart disease and may possibly protect against cancer; they define moderate drinking as one drink per day for women and two drinks per day for men.

Research studies with diabetic patients revealed that people who became diabetics at an older age and drank moderately, were 80% less likely to die from vascular heart problems.

More recent studies report that red wine had a significant effect on decreasing cholesterol, even more than vitamin E, which has long been promoted as a cholesterol-lowering nutrient. This may explain why the people of France, who eat four times more saturated fat than Americans, have fewer deaths caused by heart disease. Eighty percent of the alcohol used in France is consumed as wine, versus thirteen percent in the U.S.

Wine contains phenolic flavonoids such as quircetin and resveratrol, which function as antioxidants to protect the body cells from disease. Resveratrol (found in the skin of grapes, wine made from grapes, and grape juice) is a strong antioxidant with properties that resist fungal attack and infection. In laboratory studies, the resveratrol in wine was effective in stopping the development of cancer during the three stages of growth, and when added with quircetin, it was effective in destroying human cancer cells. Wine made from grapes appears to have added protective properties when it is compared to spirits and beer. But researchers also noted that people who reported drinking wine also reported eating more fish, fruits, vegetables, and appear to be more health conscious.

One large U.S. study among men and women with cardiovascular problems revealed that wine, spirits and beer had the same cardio-protective benefits, when consumed in moderation. In addition, people who drank with their food had an even greater benefit.

Red wine may be healthier than spirits or beer, but all the researchers do not agree. Until further research on the wine confirms the proposed benefits, we cannot say for sure that wine is better than beer or spirits, even when consumed in moderation. All researchers acknowledge that good health habits, as in reduced alcohol consumption, healthy diet, regular exercise, no smoking and maintaining ideal body weight, are all equally important for a long and healthy life. Red wine made from dark red grapes with high antioxidant content including Cabernet Sauvignon, Merlot, red Zinfandel and Petit Syrah.

The U.S. Department of Treasury approved the following statements to be used on wine labels.

1. The proud people who made this wine encourage you to consult your family doctor about the health effects of wine consumption.

2. To learn the health effects of wine consumption, send for the Federal Government's Dietary Guidelines for Americans, Center for Nutrition Policy and Promotion, USDA, 1120 20th Street N.W. Washington, DC 20036 or Visit its Website.

WHAT IS MODERATE DRINKING?

One drink for women
& Older adults
Two drinks for men

How much is one drink?

> *One drink is:*
>
> A 12-ounce glass of beer
> or
> A 5-ounce glass of wine
> or
> 1-1/2 shot distilled spirits

Who should not drink Alcohol

- *Children and teenagers*
- *A recovering alcoholic*
- *A person with family history of alcoholism*
- *A woman trying to conceive*
- *A woman who is already pregnant*
- *People who are planning to drive or operate machinery*
- *People who are taking medications*

WINES FROM GREECE

Greece is the first homeland of wine made from grapes and could have been the predominant wine producer in Europe, but the Greeks took their expertise into Rome, and it was the Roman Empire that carried the art of wine making to Northern and Western Europe. Centuries later, the Greeks have regained the respect as masters in wine making, producing excellent wines from the various mainland regions as well as the islands.

The island of Crete has been producing wine from grapes since the ancient times. Central Crete in particular, is famous for its delicious grape varieties, which ripen in September and October. The mild climate of the island is ideal for producing excellent wine, which has been praised by classical poets and writers. The red wines are dry with full body and flavor, while whites are delicately dry with a delicate aroma of white flowers and fresh fruit. One of my favorite wines from this region is called "Kretikos," produced from the Moschato grapes in Sitia, on the northeast region of the island; its fruity aromas and velvety taste make it the ideal accompaniment to fish, chicken, fruit and cheese. Other good wines from Crete include Topikos, Martiko, Logado and Myrtos. In addition, Vineyards on the west coast of Crete produce excellent wines including Kissamos in red, Asyrtiko in white and the local red table wines without the resin. The best Retsina wine in the island is produced in Hania, but it is highly resinated.

Chapter 15

Caffeine

COFFEE

Coffee is one of the world's favorite beverages originally cultivated by the Arabs for its energizing properties in 1000 A.D. Later, coffee became popular by the Italians, followed by the English and later by the French. During the seventeenth century, coffee houses in London and Paris were the popular places to "be seen." During this time, coffee was popular among intellectuals such as politicians, artists and scholars. By the eighteenth century coffee was the most popular export. From an economic point of view, the demand to please the consumer with different varieties and roasting methods has helped to maintain the economy of many third world countries.

Up to the end of the seventeenth century most of the coffee came from Arabia. Currently, half of the coffee beans we use come from Brazil, and the other half from African and Latin American countries. Today, we are the leaders in coffee consumption and the appeal for coffee in the US is unbelievable! New coffee shops open every day across the country.

The coffee plant is an evergreen and when in bloom, it is covered with little white flowers and red cherries. The plant grows best at elevations between 4,500 to 6,000 feet, and can reach forty feet in height and live more than one hundred years. During the harvest, the seed from the cherry fruit is removed, dried and roasted as the coffee bean. The roasting process determines the coffee's intensity, color and flavor. The lighter roasted coffee beans are more flavorful and contain more caffeine, and the darker roasts are roasted at higher temperatures and contain less caffeine. Although caffeine is found in many prescribed medications and over-the-counter medicines including aspirin, the caffeine in coffee is completely absorbed by the body in just a few minutes after consumption. The immediate effects of caffeine are:

- *Stimulates the nervous system*

- *Improves alertness*

- *Improves mood and stamina*

- *Decreases headaches*

- *Relaxes muscle tension*

- *Releases fat stores*

COFFEE CONSUMPTION IN RELATION TO HEALTH AND DISEASE

Because caffeine is considered a natural diuretic, consumption of coffee may lead to dehydration, if the water loss is not replaced. Constant dehydration can promote urinary stone disease, cancer of the colon, breast and urinary tract. Although some calcium is lost during dehydration, these losses are very small and can easily be replaced by eating a balanced diet. Coffee drinkers should drink additional water.

Studies funded by The American Cancer Society report "no relationship at all" between caffeine consumption and cancer, and that it may even protect against colorectal cancer. Coffee appears to improve movement and elimination of cholesterol, bile acids and metabolites that cause cancer in the colon; it contains substances that neutralize or destroy carcinogens, which are formed during cooking of meat and have been implicated for colon cancer. In addition, one out of nine women in the United States is afflicted with breast cancer, but the current research reveals no association between caffeine consumption and breast cancer.

Hypertension is another health concern, but there is no evidence that moderate coffee consumption increases the risk for this disease. However, for the people who already have hypertension, more than two cups of coffee can raise the level of cortisol (stress hormone) by constricting the blood vessels and making the heart pump harder. This results in further increase of blood pressure.

Conversely, caffeine increases muscle strength, promotes carbohydrate metabolism and relaxes the bronchial smooth muscle making it easier to breathe. The theophylline in coffee stimulates the heart and respiratory system, making caffeine effective in the treatment of asthma and allergies. If medications are not readily available, some physicians advise drinking two to three cups of coffee as another option to treatment.

Can the caffeine in coffee increase the risk of heart disease? Several recent scientific studies of women and men who drank up to five cups of coffee per day revealed no correlation between coffee consumption and heart disease. Caffeine acts as an antioxidant preventing oxidation of blood lipids, which are responsible for the formation of plaque in the artery walls.

Another important consideration is how much caffeine effects fertility and pregnancy? In one research study, women who consumed 500 mgs of caffeine a day had a more difficult time conceiving than women who did not drink coffee. As for during the gestation period, caffeine is metabolized much slower during pregnancy and can penetrate the placenta, and as the fetus is not able to metabolize caffeine, the oxygen supply to the fetus is compromised. Women who are pregnant or are trying to conceive should avoid consuming food and beverage products containing caffeine, just to be on the safe side. In addition, women who drink coffee regularly should know that coffee tends to decrease the length of the menstrual cycles, and in some women, caffeine appears to induce symptoms resembling Post Menstrual Syndrome (PMS); increased tension, irritability and anxiety, and breast tenderness.

Recent research suggests that some people become addicted to coffee and it has been an issue of concern among the medical community for many years. Some coffee drinkers find that when they deprive themselves of coffee for one to two days, they experience withdrawal symptoms, even if they normally drink one cup of coffee per day. These symptoms include decreased mental alertness, headache, nervousness, irritability and fatigue. In other people, the caffeine in coffee helps to relieve tension and headaches. New evidence suggests that caffeine combined with aspirin or ibuprofen is 40% more effective in reducing headaches, and appears to be safe and easily tolerated.

A more recent research on the effects of coffee consumption showed that it helps protect the gallbladder from bacterial infection by improving movement of digestive substances. Thus, caffeine helps protect against the formation of gallstones, a disease affecting over twenty million people in the U.S. Gallstones are formed in the body when bile containing a lot of cholesterol becomes insoluble and forms stones, clogging the bile ducts of pancreas and forming bacteria, which leads to infection. Bacterial infection may spread to other parts of the body.

Overall, coffee is considered a harmless beverage. The popularity of coffee is mainly due to its short-

term benefits and minor side effects. There is very little evidence that moderate intake of coffee relates to illness, on the other hand, there is considerable evidence to support consuming coffee as a benefit to health.

SUGGESTIONS FOR COFFEE DRINKERS

Use unbleached coffee filters, and limit consumption to two cups per day.

Try the lighter more robust beans. Lighter roasts contain more caffeine, but are less carcinogenic.

Organic blends of coffee are safer. Coffee from tropical regions may contain chemical pesticides.

If you drink decaffeinated coffee, use only water processed decaffeinated coffee.

Try drinking Green tea instead of regular coffee.

Women who experience symptoms of PMS should reduce the amount of caffeine they drink during this period.

TEA

Tea is one of the world's oldest beverages, dating back to 2737 B.C., and has been China's national drink since the sixth century. For thousands of years people believed that tea offers many health benefits. By the sixteenth century, tea was traded between the East and West. "Taking Tea" was a custom that began in East India, and practiced in

Hong Kong and Great Britain. The Scottish began the practice of "High Tea", which was served between five and six o'clock in the late afternoon, often accompanied by sausage or egg pie.

When tea was first discovered, it was very expensive and therefore, it was considered the beverage of the rich. Later, the consumption of tea became an important part of culture in the United Kingdom, Ireland, India, China, Japan and other Asian countries. The English liked tea so much that they adopted it as their national drink, with the average person drinking over three cups per day. In the U.S., the popularity of tea is very recent due to the plethora of tea varieties offered and aggressive advertising by the tea industry. The majority of the Americans drink iced tea regularly, and due to their influence on other countries, iced tea is now popular in Europe.

Camellia sinensis, the true tea plant, grows best in tropical and subtropical climates. Every year, two and a half million tons of tea is produced from the camellia sinensis plant. China and Japan are the primary tea producers. Higher altitudes and tropical climates produce higher quality crops. The best tea is produced from young and unopened leaf buds. These young buds contain a lot of caffeine and phytochemicals, which have been found to promote good health.

The camellia sinensis plant produces three different kinds of tea: black, green and oolong. 80% of the total consumption of tea is produced as black tea and is preferred variety in Europe, India and North America. The remaining 20% is produced as oolong and green tea, which are preferred varieties in Asia. Popular herb teas like berry blends, mint, chamomile, cinnamon and other fruit flavor teas are not considered true teas. Herb teas may have some flavonoids, but do not have the same antioxidant benefit as true tea.

Research shows that true tea helps lower heart disease, cancer and other illnesses, especially green tea. The flavanol, Epigallocatechin Gallate (EGCG), a stronger antioxidant in green tea, is one hundred times more powerful than vitamin C, twenty-five times more powerful than vitamin E and twice as effective as the phenols in red wine. Animal studies on the affects of tea on health are very encouraging. While green tea is effective in fighting against diseases due to its more powerful antioxidant properties, black and oolong tea have protective properties as well.

Overall, most scientific studies show that true tea appears to inhibit the initiation and promotion of cancer cells, in addition to other health benefits. Animal studies have shown positive results, but human studies are conflicting. Hopefully, human studies in the future will have similar results. There is very little evidence that tea is not beneficial to health, and the benefits of drinking tea appear to outweigh the risks.

THE BENEFITS OF DRINKING TEA

- Green tea may help reduce swelling associated with arthritis.
- Black and green tea may lower the risk of pancreatic and prostate cancer.
- Green tea improves the body's ability to fight the flu virus.
- Green tea kills bacteria in the mouth that cause cavities.
- Green tea helps neutralize enzymes found in bacteria and viruses, and stops tumor cells from growing.
- Oolong tea extract has shown to be effective in reducing plaque on teeth.
- May protect against breast cancer during stages one and two.
- May reduce risk of heat attack.

SUGGESTIONS FOR TEA DRINKERS

Store the tea bags or loose tea in an airtight container to preserve the potency and flavor.

Steep the tea in hot water for five minutes before drinking to maximize the flavonoid content.

Because the flavonoid content in tea interferes with the absorption of iron, avoid eating iron-containing foods when drinking tea.

True teas include the black tea varieties such as Earl Grey, English or Irish Breakfast and Darjeeling.

Glossary

Absorption is the transfer of nutrients across the cell membrane. After the digestion of food, the nutrients are transferred from the intestines to the blood and lymph circulation to be absorbed.

Aerobic is the requirement of oxygen by living organism.

Amino Acids are organic acids containing an amino nitrogen group, which is essential in building protein chains.

Anaerobic is the absence of oxygen in living things.

Anemia is a deficiency of red blood cells or packed cell volume.

Anorexia is a loss of appetite.

Anorexia Nervosa is an intentional dangerous underweight condition requiring professional treatment.

Anthocyanins are a pigment in blue-red fruits, which fight against cancer.

Antibody is a protein of the blood produced in response to an invasion from a foreign organism or the presence of bacteria.

Antioxidant is a substance that prevents deterioration by preventing oxidation; it reacts with oxygen to protect other compounds from oxygen.

Atherosclerosis is a disease caused by an accumulation of fatty deposits in the artery walls, causing loss of elasticity and hardening of the arteries.

Bile is a substance made from cholesterol by the liver and it is stored in the gallbladder.

Biological value (BV) is a measure for protein quality determined by how well a particular protein supports nitrogen retention.

Calcification is the hardening of bone tissue by a deposit of calcium, as well as magnesium salts.

Capsaicin is a potent antioxidant in hot peppers.

Collagen is a protein that makes up the bone matrix, connective tissue and cartilage.

Complete Protein is a protein containing all the essential amino acids needed for human growth and development.

Coronary relates to the blood vessels supplying the heart.

Dehydration is a dangerous condition, when the body responds to excessive water losses.

Detoxify to remove or withdraw harmful toxins.

Digestion is the breakdown of foods by hydrolysis in the digestive tract to smaller substances that can be used by the body.

Diuretic is a substance that causes increased water excretion.

Edamane is an unshelled fresh soybean pod.

"Empty calories" are foods containing calories, but only small amounts from nutrients.

Emulsifier is a compound with water-soluble and fat-soluble properties that can attract fat to water-soluble solutions.

Essential amino acid is an amino acid that cannot be synthesized sufficiently to meet our physiological needs and must be supplied by the diet.

Glossary

Essential fatty acid is one that must be present in the diet to prevent deficiencies of nutrients.

Fat is a lipid that is solid at room temperature.

Fluid balance refers to an even fluid distribution throughout the body tissues and compartments.

Fortification is the addition of nutrients to regularly consumed foods to prevent deficiencies of important nutrients.

Frame size refers to the size of a persons bones and musculature.

Glucose is a single sugar present in fruits and honey, or obtained from the breakdown complex carbohydrates.

Hunger is a physiological response to a need for food.

Junk food refers to foods containing high amounts of salt, sugar, or fat.

Ideal body weight is the average weight given by statistical data according to the national average for the healthiest population. It may not be ideal for a given individual.

Insulin is a hormone secreted by the pancreas to promote the utilization of glucose in an effort to lower the level of glucose in the blood.

Lactobacillus is a favorable bacteria substance in yogurt that reacts as an antioxidant to protect body cells.

Lipogenesis is the formation of fat.

Low-density lipoproteins are complexes of cholesterol, lipids, proteins and triglycerides in the blood.

Lycopene is the red pigment in tomatoes and a powerful substance in destroying cancers cells.

Metabolism is the chemical and physical processes occurring within the organism by utilizing and breaking-down protein, fat and sugar substances to produce energy.

Nausea is the inclination to vomit, induced by illness of the stomach.

Nutrients density is the high ratio of nutrient content in food in proportion to the amount of calories.

Omega-3 fatty acids are long chained polyunsaturated fats found in the oils of fish and shellfish.

Osteoporosis is the reduction of bone tissue from calcium deficiency.

Osteomalacia is softening of the bones caused by calcium and vitamin D deficiencies.

Polyphenols are antioxidants found in green tea that help prevent the growth of cancer cells.

Salmonella is a bacteria causing intestinal infection in humans.

Satiety is the feeling of satisfaction or fullness after eating.

Sulforaphane is an anti-cancerous substance found in broccoli.

Triglycerides are fats made by the body from the foods we eat; they are carried in the blood and stored as body fat.

References

PROFESSIONAL JOURNALS:

Adams, AK. EO Wermuth and PE McBride. *Antioxidant vitamins and the prevention of coronary heart disease*, American Family Physician, 60:895-904,1999

Allison D.B, et al. *Annual deaths attributable to obesity in the United States* JAMA, 282: 1530-38, 1999.

Astrup, A., et al. *The role of low-fat diets and fat substitutes in body weight management: What have we learned from clinical studies?* Journal of the American Dietetic Association, 97: S82-S87, 1997.

Barrett BB et al. *Assessing The Risks And Benefits Of Herbal Medicine: An Overview Of Scientific Evidence*, Alternative Therapies, 5: 40-49, 1999.

Barrett BB et al. *Echinacea for upper respiratory infections* Journal of Family Practice, 39: 425-16, 1999.

Bar-o, M. E. *The effects of television on child health: implications and recommendations* Arch Dis in Child, 83: 289-92, 2000.

Bay, G.A. *Obesity: A time bomb to be defused.* Lancet 352:160-61, 1998

Berger A. *Why Wine Might Be Less Harmful Than Beer And Spirits.* British Medical Journal, 317:848, 1998

Birch LL and J.O. Fisher. *Development of eating behaviors among children and adolescents* Pediatrics, 101: 539-48, 1998

Bonnelli L. et al. *Coffee consumption and pancreatic cancer: A cancer-controlled case-control study (reply).* European Journal of Gastroenterology and Hepatology, 6: 190-9, 1994

Bull FC, Jamrozik K. *Advice on exercise from a family physician can help sedentary patients to become more active.* American Journal of Preventive Medicine, 15: 85-94, 1998

Coulston, A.M. *Obesity as an epidemic:* Facing the Challenge Journal of the American Dietetic Association, 98:S6-S8, 1998

Dietary Guidelines For Americans, United States Department of Agriculture; 1995

Dietz W. H. *Critical periods in childhood for the development of obesity* American Journal Of Clinical Nutrition, 59: 955-9, 1994.

Dietz W. H. *Health consequences of obesity in youth: childhood predictors of adult disease* Pediatrics 101: 518-514,1998

Eisenberg DM et al. *Trends In Alternative Medicine Use In The United States, 1990-1997* Journal of the American Medical Association, 280:1569-75, 1998

Emmert, DH and JT Kirchner. *The role of vitamin E in the prevention of heart disease,* Archives of Family Medicine, 8(6): 537-542,1999

Epstien L.H. et al. *Problem solving in the treatment of childhood obesity* Journal of Consulting in Clinical Psychology, 68: 717-21, 2000

Eskenazi B et al. *Associations between maternal decaffeinated and caffeinated coffee consumption, and fetal growth and gestation duration,* Epidemiology, 10: 242-49, 1999

Fenster L et al. Caffeine consumption and menstrual function, American Journal of Epidemiology, 149: 550-57, 1999

Fenster L. et al. *Caffeinated beverages decaffeinated coffee consumption and spontaneous abortion.* Epidemiology, 8: 515-22,1997

Flora K et al. *Milk thistle (silybum marianum) for the therapy of liver disease,* American Journal of Gastroenterology, 93: 139-43, 1998

Hill, J.O. and J.C. Peters. *Environmental contributions to the obesity epidemic* Science, 280:1471-4, 1998

Hillbom M, Juvela S. Alcohol And Risk For Stroke. *Alcohol and The Cardiovascular Syste*m: Research Monograph No. 31. Bethesda MD: National Institute of Health, 63-83, 1996

Holman, Rt. *The slow discovery of the importance of omega 3 essential fatty acids in human health,* Journal of Nutrition, 128 (suppl2): 427S-433S, 1998

Holman, RT. The slow discovery of the importance of omega 3 essential fatty acids in human health, Journal of Nutrition, 128(Suppl 2): 427S-433S, 1998

Horswill CA. *Effective fluid replacement*, International Journal of Sports Nutrition, 8: 175-95, 1998

Innes G. *Cost-effectiveness of beer versus red wine for the prevention of symptomatic coronary artery disease*, Canadian Medical Association Journal, 159: 1463-6, 1998

Jequier, E. and L. Tappy. *Regulation of body weight in humans* Physiology Review, 79:451-80,1999

Kampman E, et al. *Calcium, Vitamin D, Dairy Foods and The Occurrence Of Colorectal Adenomas Among Men and Women in Two Prospective Studies*, American Journal of Epidemiology, 38: 16-29, 1994

Klatsky Al, et al. *Red Wine, White Wine, Liquor And Risk For Coronary Artery Disease Hospitalization.* American Journal of Cardiology 80: 416-20, 1997

Kleiner S. Water: *An Essential Overlooked Nutrient.* Journal of the American Dietetic Association, 99: 200-06, 1999

Kuczmarshi, R.J., et al. *Increasing prevalence of overweight among U.S adults.* JAMA, 282:1579-80, 1994

Lonnqvist, F., Nordfors, L. and M. Schalling. *Leptin and its potential role in human obesity.* J Intern Med, 245:643.

Maffeis C. et al *Distribution of food intake as a risk factor for childhood obesity* Int J Obes, 24 :75-80, 2000

Marchmann, P and M Gronbaek. *Fish consumption and coronary heart disease mortality: A systematic review of prospective cohort studies*, European Journal of Clinical Nutrition, 53(8): 585-590, 1999

Martinez M.A., et al. Association of Diet and Colorectal Adenomatous Polyps: Dietary Fiber, Calcium, and Total Fat. Epidemiology, **7**: 264-68, 1996

Marinades may drastically decrease cancer risk posed by grilling. *Press Release*. American Institute for Cancer Research. June 18, 1999

McCrory, M.A., et al. *Overeating in America: Association between restaurant consumption and body fatness in healthy adult men and women ages 19 to 80*   Obesity Research,   7:564-71 1999

Mokdad, A.H., et al. *The spread of the obesity epidemic in the United States:* 1991-1998.   JAMA, 282: 1519-22,1999

Mylonas, C and D Kouretas. *Lipid per oxidation and tissue damage,* In Vitro, 13 (3): 295-309,1999

National Coffee Association: The History of Coffee. www.ncausa.org

National Institute of Environmental Health Sciences: The truth about caffeine, National Institute of Health. (www.niehs.nih.gov/odhsb/focus/summer97/caffeine.html

Nehlig A. *Are We Dependent Upon Coffee and Caffeine? A Review on Human and Animal* Data   Neuroscience and bio-behavioral Reviews, 23: 563-76, 1999

Nehlig A., Debry G. Coffee and Cancer: A Review of Human and Animal Data. World Review of Nutrition and Dietetics, 79: 185-221, 1996

Nieves J.W., et al. Calcium Potentials: *The Effect of Estrogen and Calcitonin on Bone Mass: Review and Analysis.* American Journal of Clinical Nutrition, 67: 18-24, 1998

O'Hara MA et al. A Review Of 12 Commonly Used Medicinal Herbs Archives of Family Medicine, 7: 523-36, 1998

Oken BS. et al. *The efficacy of ginkgo biloba on cognitive function in Alzheimer disease,* Archives of Neurology, 55: 1409-13, 1998

O'Mathuna DP. *Goldenseal: The golden cure to common colds?* Alternative Medicine Alert, 1:90-93, 1998

Renaud S. de Logeril M. Wine, alcohol, platelets, and the French Paradox for coronary heart disease. The Lancet, 339: 1523-26,1992.

Rogers P. Dernoncourt C. *Regular Caffeine Consumption: A Balance of Adverse and Beneficial Effects for Mood and Psychomotor Performance.*   Pharmacology Biochemistry and Behavior, 59: 1039-45, 1998

Moderate Drinking. *Alcohol Alert.* #16. National Institute On Alcohol Abuse And Alcoholism. April 1992

Rippe, M.M. and S. Hess. *The Role of physical activity in the prevention and management of obesity,* Journal of the American Dietetic Association, 98: S31-S38, 1998

Robinson, T.N., et al. *Reducing children's television viewing to prevent obesity: A randomized controlled trial.* JAMA, 282: 1561-1567, 1999

Sikora R et al. *Ginkgo biloba extract in the therapy of erectile dysfunction,* Journal of Urology, 141: 188A, 1989

Simopoulos, AP. *Essential fatty acids in health and chronic disease,* American Journal of Clinical Nutrition, 70:(Suppl): 560S-569S, 1999

Story, M, et al. *Dieting status and its relationship to eating and physical activity behaviors in a representative sample of US adolescents.* Journal of the American Dietetics Association, 98:1127-1132, 1998

Sesso H. et al. *Coffee and Tea Intake and The Risk Of Myocardial Infarction,* American Journal of Epidemiology, 149: 162-67, 1999

Tavani A et al. *Coffee consumption and the risk of breast cancer,* European Journal of Cancer Prevention, 7:77-82, 1998

The History of Tea (www.stashtea.com)

Tea Council. Tea and health (www.teacouncil.co.uk)

Teen Alcohol Consumption: American Academy of Pediatrics Survey; Summary of Findings. September 30, 1998

Tepper BJ. Nayga Jr. RM *Awareness of the link between bone disease and calcium intake is associated with higher dietary calcium intake in women aged 50 years and older:* report of the 1991 CSFII-DHKS. Journal of The American Dietetic Association, 98: 196-98, 1998

Thune I., et al. Physical activity and the risk of breast cancer, New England Journal of Medicine 336: 1269-75, 1997

Treasury Announces Actions Concerning Labeling Of Alcoholic Beverages, *Office of Public Affairs, U.S. Department of treasury.* February 5, 1999

Tribble, DL. *Antioxidant consumption and risk of coronary heart disease: emphasis on vitamin C, Vitamin E and B-carotene,* Circulation, 99:591-595, 1999

Troiano, R.P. and K.M. Flegal. *Overweight prevalence among youth in the United States: Why so many different numbers?* Int J Obesity 23: S22-S27, 1999

Vale S. *Subarachnoid hemorrhage associated with Ginkgo biloba* Lancet 352:36, 1998

Van Mil, E.G., et al. *Physical activity and the prevention of childhood obesity-Europe versus the United States* Int J Obesity 23: S41-S4, 1999

Willett W et al. *Coffee Consumption and Coronary Heart Disease in Women.* Journal of the American Medical Association 2756:458-62, 1996

Williams GD et al. Apparent Per Capita Alcohol Consumption: National, State, And Regional Trends, 1977-96. Surveillance Report: #47. National Institute on Alcohol Abuse and Alcoholism. December 1998

Books

Height & Weight Tables, Metropolitan Life Insurance Company, New York, NY, 1999

Brownell, K.D. The LEARN Program for Weight Control, seventh edition. Dallas, TX: American Health Publishing company, 1997

Carlson, Wade. Eat Away Illness, Parker Publishing, West Nyack, New York, 1986
Clark N. Nancy Clark's Sports Nutrition Handbook, second edition Champaign, IL. Human Kinetics, 1997

Cotton, R.T., Editor. Personal Trainer Manual, San Diego, CA: American Council on Exercise, 1996

Coleman E, Steen SN. The Ultimate Sports Nutrition Handbook Palo Alto, CA: Bull Publishing, 1996

References

Edwards B. <u>America's Favorite Drug:</u> *Coffee and Your Health.* Berkeley, CA: <u>Odonian Press</u>, 1992.

Marshall, W. Charles <u>Vitamins and Minerals</u> George F. Stickley, Philadelphia, PA. 1983

Mellin, L. <u>The Solution: 6 ways to Permanent Weight Loss</u>, New York, NY: Regan Books, 1997

Normandi, C.E. and L. Roark <u>It's Not About Food,</u> New York, NY: Grosset Putman, 1998

Peeke, Pamela <u>Fight Fat After Forty</u> Penguin Books, New York, N.Y., 2001

<u>Physicians' Desk Reference</u>, fifty-third Edition. New Jersey: Medical Economics Data, 1999

<u>Prevent Disease, Achieve Maximum Physical Performance,</u> New York, NY: Harper Collins, 1995

Rodale's Illustrated Encyclopedia of Herbs, 1987

<u>Seafood Resource for Educators:</u> National Fisheries Education and Research Foundation Washington, D.C.

Gussow, J.D. and Thomas P.R. <u>The Nutrition Debate</u>: Bull Publishing; Polo Alto, CA., 1986

U.S. Department of Health and Human Services <u>Physical Activity and Health: A Report of the Surgeon General,</u> Atlanta, GA: USDIIHS and center for Disease Control and Prevention, 1996

World Health Organization, <u>Obesity: Preventing and Managing the Global Epidemic,</u> Geneva: World Health Organization, 1998

INDEX

Aerobic, 92, 93
Aging, 55
Alcohol, 223-229
Allergies, 57
Amino acids, 43
Anaerobic, 92, 93
Anorexia Nervosa,
Antioxidants, 52
Arteriosclerosis, 6
Bile,
Balance diet, 39,58,59
BMR, 37-39
Body fat, 1,2
Capsaicin, 69
Caffeine, 230-238
Calcium, 19-25
Calcification, 240
Calories, 38
Cancer, 5
Cholesterol, 6, 44, 45
Collagen, 240
Coronary disease, 6
Crustaceans, 111
Diabetes, 8
Diuretic, 9
Cooking Herbs, 102-109
Danger Zone, 110
Diet Recommendations;
   For children, 34
   For teenagers, 36
   For adults, 74
Energy needs, 37, 99
   Calories, 37, 99, 4 0, 43, 44
   Carbohydrates, 40
   Protein, 43
Epinephrine, 39
Essential amino acids,
Fats, 44
   Monounsaturated, 45
   Polyunsaturated, 44
   Saturated, 44
   Omega-3 fatty acids, 44
Fiber, 54
Food born illness, 110
Food Portions, 76-89
Food Portion Charts,
Glucose, 40-43
Glycogen, 42
Height & Weigh Charts
   For women, 97
   For men, 98
Herbal Remedies, 212
   Blue Cohosh, 219
   Chamomile, 214
   Comfrey, 219
   Deadly Nightshade, 219
   Echinacea, 214
   Ephedra, 219
   Feverfew, 215
   Foxglove, 219
   Ginseng, 215
   Ginkgo Biloba, 216
   Gordenseal, 216
   Jimsonweed, 219
   Juniper, 219
   Life Root, 219
   Lobelia , 220
   Saw Palmetto, 217
   Kava-kava, 217
   Milk Thistle, 217
   Mistletoe, 221
   Pokeroot, 221
   Sassafras, 221
   St. John's-wort, 218
   Tropical Periwinkle, 220
   Valerian Root, 217
HDL, 6, 45
Insulin, 3, 8, 42, 43
Lactobacillus, 71
LDL, 6, 44
Lycopene, 70
Meal Plan, 74
Mollusks, 111
Minerals & Trace Elements, 48
   Calcium, 19-25, 49
   Chromium, 51
   Cobalt, 51
   Copper, 51
   Fluoride, 51
   Iodine, 51
   Iron, 49
   Magnesium, 50
   Phosphorus, 49
   Potassium, 50
   Selenium, 50
   Sodium, 51
   Zinc, 49
Metabolism, 38
Nutrient, 37
Nutrient dense, 37
Obesity, 1-4, 27-31
Olive oil, 68, 106

Omega-3, 44
Osteoporosis, 16
Phytochemicals, 52
Phenolic Flavonoids, 242
Relaxation, 95
Resveratrol, 226
Salmonella, 113
Sulforaphane, 65
Safe food handling, 111
   Seafood, 111
   Chicken, 113
   Eggs, 113
Snacks, 62
Tea, 252-254
Triglycerides, 44, 242
Vitamins;
   Vitamin A, 45, 55, 56, 57
      Source of,
         Beta-carotene, 45, 70
   Vitamin B;
      Folic Acid, 46
      Niacin, 46
      Pyridoxine, 46
      Riboflavin, 47
      Thiamin, 46
      Cobalamin, 46
   Vitamin C, 71, 72, 73, 47
   Vitamin D, 47
   Vitamin E, 48
   Vitamin K, 48

COOKBOOK

Starters

Bean Soup, 129
Cheese Puff, 131
Cheese Spread with Smoked
      Salmon, 141
Chicken Salad, 125
Chicken Soup, 127
Egg Whites Stuffed
      with Liver Pate, 133
Eggplant Salad, 123
Greek Salad, 119
Hardy white Bread, 116
Lentil Soup, 126
Pita Bread, 117
Pepper & Peach Salad, 120
Potato Salad, 124
Potato Clam Soup, 130
Red Roasted Peppers Stuffed with
    Cheese, 140

Cheese Spread with Smoked
      Samon, 141
Sautéed Calamari, 134
Sautéed Meatballs, 135
Stuffed Grape Leaves, 137
Village Salad, 121
Winter Salad, 122
Yellow Split Pea Spread, 139
Yogurt & Cucumber Sauce, 138
Zucchini Croquettes, 136
Zucchini Omelet, 118

Vegetarian Dishes

Artichokes & Potatoes in Lemon, 149
Baked Beans, 151
Black-eyed peas with Rice, 145
Butter Beans with Dill, 161
Garlic Mashed Potatoes, 150
Green Beans with Tomatoes
    & Herbs, 146
Fettuccini with Garlic & Basil, 147
Eggplant Vinaigrette, 154
Pita stuffed with Avocado Salad, 147
Potatoes with Oregano & Lemon, 161
Potatoes & Green Peas, 160
Portabella Mushroom Sandwich, 144
Risotto with Spinach, 148
Rice Pilaf, 152
Seared Vegetables, 152
Spinach & Cheese Pie, 158
Spinach With Peppers & Almonds, 155
Steamed Greens, 153
Tomatoes Stuffed with Rice
    & Herbs, 156

Meat & Poultry

Braised Lamb in Red Wine Sauce, 164
Baked Italian Meatballs, 168
Baked Ziti with Meat Sauce, 170
Beef Burritos with Green Chile
    Sauce, 174
Chicken Enchiladas, 172
Green Chile Sauce, 173
Lamb Chops with Mushrooms
    & Mint, 171
Lamb with Rice Pine Nuts
    & Raisins, 165
Oriental Chicken & Shrimp, 175
Pork Tenderloin with Apples &
    Apricots, 167
Roast Chicken & Potatoes, 176

Index

Roast Cornish Hens with Apples & Raisins, 177
Roast Lamb & Potatoes, 166
Spanish Salsa, 171
Veal Scaloppini, 169

Seafood

Baked Clams, 180
Baked Filet of Halibut, 183
Baked Salmon, 187
Baked Trout, 192
Belgium Endives Stuffed with Salmon, 188
Chilled Shrimp & Crab Salad, 182
Filet of Sole with Almonds, 183
Mussels in Red Wine Sauce, 185
Salmon glazed with Honey & Almonds, 189
Sea-bass & Scallops in Wine Sauce, 191
Seafood Chowder, 186

The Sweet Shop

Apples Baked in Phyllo Pastry, 199
Baklava, 194
Banana Zucchini Bread, 209
Bread Pudding, 205
Butter Cookies, 196
Crepes with Yogurt & Raspberries, 206
Donut Puffs, 207
Easter Bread, 208
Honey Macaroons, 197
New Year's Day Cake, 210
Rice Pudding, 200
Spanish Custard, 201
Semolina Custard with Raspberries, 202
Walnut Cake, 203
Yogurt Cake, 204

Quick Order Form

Postal Orders: Copper Hill Press
Post Office Box 13628
Tucson, Arizona 85732-3628
520-886-9800

Website: http://www.copperhillpress.com

Fax Orders: 520-290-5657

Name: _____

Address: _____

Telephone _____

E-Mail: _____

"Healthy Living From A Greek Island"

Book Price in the U.S	$34.95
Shipping and Handling:	$6.95
Arizona Residents Please Add 5% Tax	_____
Total Amount Enclosed:	_____

Credit Card: _____Visa _____MC

Credit Card Number: _____

Expiration Date: _____

Signature: _____

Quick Order Form

Postal Orders: Copper Hill Press
Post Office Box 13628
Tucson, Arizona 85732-3628
520-886-9800
Website: http://www.copperhillpress.com

Fax Orders: 520-290-5657

Name: _____

Address: _____

Telephone _____

E-Mail: _____

"Healthy Living From A Greek Island"

Book Price in the U.S.: $34.95

Shipping and Handling: $6.95

Arizona Residents Please Add
5% Tax   _____

Total Amount Enclosed: _____

Credit Card: _____Visa _____MC

Credit Card Number: _____

Expiration Date: _____

Signature: _____